# Essential Oils

and

# Therapeutic Blends

in Colour

# Essential Oils
## and
# Therapeutic Blends
## in Colour

## Essential Oils for 50 Common Ailments

### by
# Rosemary Caddy

First paperback edition 2023

Book design by PublishingPush

Paperback ISBN: 978-1-80541-014-0
eBook ISBN: 978-1-80541-015-7

# About the Author

Rosemary Caddy, BSc Hons, ARCS, MISPA

Rosemary Caddy graduated from London University with a BSc Honours Degree in Science. As a Reader and Principal Lecturer in Educational Research at Nottingham University she is the author of a range of educational materials for students of many disciplines. All the materials emphasise visual presentation to enable students to see, analyse and understand the world around them. The format of this work ranges from books to interactive video tapes and compact discs. Rosemary is now a qualified clinical aromatherapist running her own clinic and carrying out a programme of research on the chemistry of essential oils. She runs lecture courses for aromatherapy students to help them understand and visualise their essential oils. The Caddy Classic Profiles, developed as a result of her research enable students to enjoy the chemistry of their oils. Currently Rosemary is research-ing the chemistry of synergistic mixes of essential oils.

## Note to the Reader

Whilst the author has made every effort to ensure that the contents of this book are accurate in every particular, it is not intended to be regarded as a substitute for professional medical advice under treatment. The reader is urged to give careful consideration to any difficulties which he or she is experiencing with their own health and to consult their General Practitioner if uncertain as to its cause or nature. Neither the author nor the publisher can accept any legal responsibility for any health problem which results from the use of the self-help methods described.

# Acknowledgements

My interest in essential oils derives from personal experience of their powerful therapeutic properties, both in treating physical ailments and also in calming emotional problems.

Exploring the chemistry of essential oils gives some insights as to why the oils are so powerful.

My background in lecturing and research has been focused on using strong visual stumuli to communicate complex structures. Colour and pictures are excellent learning aids. Caddy Classic Profiles have been created to help communicate the nature of essential oils.

I would like to sincerely thank the following people who have contributed to this book in a variety of ways: John Ensall for his support since the early days to develop my ideas and for generous sharing of chemical data; Elaine Price of the Montrose School of Massage and Aromatherapy who recognised the work in its early stages and encouraged me to write the book offering many valuable suggestions; Katja Svoboda and her team at The Scottish Agricultural College for assistance in research into essential oils and their synergistic mixes.

I would also like to thank all my friends, family, colleagues and students who listened to all my enthusiasms so patiently. In particular special thanks to Peter, my husband, for his unflagging support and for his painstaking editing of manuscript and indices.

My appreciation also goes to the services of Nottingham and Exeter University Libraries, The British Library, The Royal Horticultural Society, Oxford Botanical Gardens and to my own local Dartmouth Library. It is my hope that this book will offer the opportunity to the reader to build an understanding of each essential oil in a pleasurable but powerful way.

# Caddy Classic Profiles

Each essential oil has its own aroma and its own unique chemical make-up. There are many books that detail the reported therapeutic properties of each oil and these reports are a good guide when deciding which oils will help a specific condition.

Part One of this book lists the reported therapeutic properties of 90 essential Oils. It also illustrates the chemical make-up of each oil by a brightly coloured piechart called a Caddy Classic Profile (CCP).

This chart shows the amount of each of the major chemical families that are typically present in each essential oil. They provide a clear fingerprint for each oil that conveys the chemical nature of the oil. In Part Two we show the CCP for 50 Therapeutic Blends.

## *Major Chemical Families*

Here we give a brief description of the chemical families that are shown in a CCP. The table below shows the colour coding used in a CCP and lists a few of the possible therapeutic properties that the chemical families may contribute to an essential oil.

| | | |
|---|---|---|
| ■ | esters | calming good for skin problems |
| ■ | aliphatic aldehydes | refreshing, antiseptic, antifungal |
| ■ | ketones | cooling, decongestant, analgesic |
| ■ | sesquiterpenes | balancing, soothing, digestion, warming |
| ■ | lactones & coumarins | balancing, decongestant, photosensitive |
| ■ | remainder | the unreported part of the oil i.e. the remainder |
| ■ | oxides | expectorant, respiratory decongestant, diuretic |
| ■ | acids | deodourant, present in very small quantities |
| ■ | aromatic aldehydes | warming, antiseptic, antifungal |
| ■ | monoterpenes | skin tonic, digestion, liver |
| ■ | alcohols | antiviral, bactericidal, tonic but gentle |
| ■ | phenols, phe. ethers | stimulating, antiviral, aggressive |

If you see a large amount of the ester blue colour you know that the oil is rich in esters. This alerts you to the fact that this oil may well help skin conditions so you check its reported properties to see if that is indeed so.

If you see a large amount of the light blue ketone colour, showing that the oil is rich in ketones, you are alerted to the fact that caution may be required in the use of this oil as ketones can accumulate in the body. Again check the properties of the oil to see if this is so.

An alert is also given when you see a large area of the dark red showing that the oil is rich in phenols. This chemical family can be highly aggressive so once more check the properties of the oil as reported in the literature.

Alcohols and esters are nearly always safe and gentle in use. Thus knowing the chemical make-up of an oils alerts you to possibilities for its therapeutic properties. However you must always refer to the reported properties of the oil to check out these possibilities. This is because each essential oil is unique in its chemical make-up. The particular set of molecules present forms the whole oil and it is the property of the whole oil that is important.

## *The Caddy Classic Profile (CCP)*

The CCP gives the typical chemical nature of an oil at a glance and allows you to quickly compare it with other essential oils.

Imagine that a chemist reports that he has found an essential oil that is really remarkable in that it typically contains all the chemical families and each one is 8% of the oil. Its CCP would be:

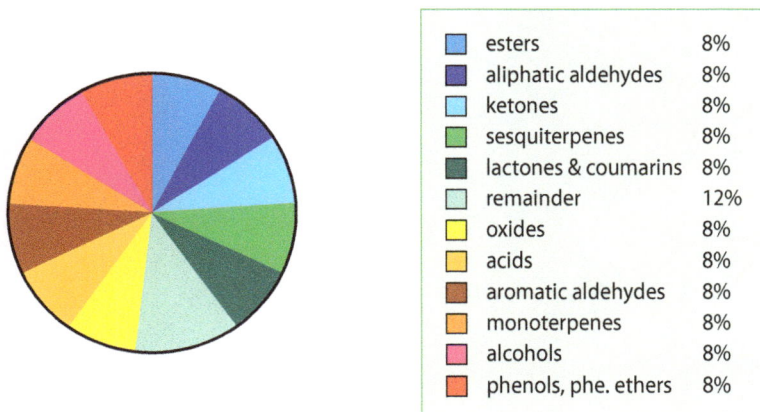

| | | |
|---|---|---|
| | esters | 8% |
| | aliphatic aldehydes | 8% |
| | ketones | 8% |
| | sesquiterpenes | 8% |
| | lactones & coumarins | 8% |
| | remainder | 12% |
| | oxides | 8% |
| | acids | 8% |
| | aromatic aldehydes | 8% |
| | monoterpenes | 8% |
| | alcohols | 8% |
| | phenols, phe. ethers | 8% |

When an oil is analysed it is expensive to identify every single chemical constituent – usually an oil distributor requests identification of the most important chemicals. The chemist in this example has identified 88% of the oil so there is still 12% of the oil's chemical constituents unidentified. This 12% remainder is shown in light green. The colours used in the CCPs give you an immediate view of the electrochemical nature of each *BLEND*. The 'blue' families share a molecular structure such that they generate negatively charged particles and the 'yellow to red' families share a molecular structure such that they generate positive particles. This tends to show up in the fact that except for a few exceptions *BLENDS* with large areas of 'blues' tend to be more relaxing, those with large areas of 'yellows to reds' tend to be more stimulating and the 'greens' are more associated with balancing properties.

# Contents

## Part One: 90 Essential Oils

## *Part Two: 50 Therapeutic Blends for 50 Common Ailments*

# Part One

---

# 90 Essential Oils

# AMYRIS
## Amyris balsamifera

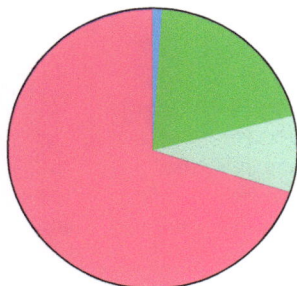

| | | |
|---|---|---|
| 🟦 | esters | 1.0% |
| 🟪 | aliphatic aldehydes | yes |
| 🟩 | sesquiterpenes | 20.0% |
| 🟩 | lactones & coumarins | yes |
| ⬜ | remainder | 9.0% |
| 🟥 | alcohols | 70.0% |

## BODY SYSTEMS

**NERVOUS SYSTEM**
🟦🟪🟩🟩

**ENDOCRINE SYSTEM**
🟥

**CIRCULATION AND IMMUNE SYSTEM**
🟦🟪🟩🟩🟥

**SKIN, MUSCLES AND BODY TISSUES**
🟦🟪🟩🟩🟥

**RESPIRATORY SYSTEM**
🟪🟩🟥

**DIGESTIVE SYSTEM**
🟦🟪🟩🟩

**URINARY SYSTEM**
🟪🟩🟥

**REPRODUCTIVE SYSTEM**
🟪🟩🟥

## PROPERTIES > USES

antispasmodic, calming >

warming >

antiviral, bactericidal, lowers blood pressure, decongestant > haemorrhoids, stimulates immune system, varicose veins

antiinflammatory, antiseptic > especially good for muscle cramps, rashes

bactericidal > bronchitis

calming > spasms

antiseptic > infections

antiseptic > infections

## BOTANICAL FAMILY

Rutaceae: this family generally aids digestion and skin problems.

Tree: distilled wood and branches : musty wood aroma : base note.
Sometimes called West Indian Sandalwood or Rosewood which can lead to confusion. It grows in abundance in Haiti and is often called 'candlewood' as its twigs make excellent torches.

Chemical constituents may include:

🟩 caryophyllene, cadinene
🟩 amyrolin

⬜ furfural
🟥 cadinol, balsamiol

3

# BASIL EUGENOL
## Ocimum gratissimum eugenoliferum

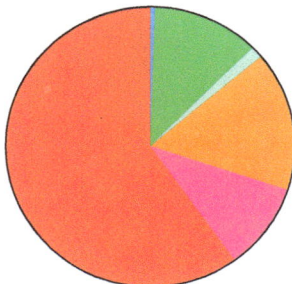

| | | |
|---|---|---|
| ■ | esters | 0.6% |
| ■ | sesquiterpenes | 12.0% |
| ■ | remainder | 1.4% |
| ■ | monoterpenes | 16.0% |
| ■ | alcohols | 10.0% |
| ■ | phenols, phe. ethers | 60.0% |

## BODY SYSTEMS

NERVOUS SYSTEM
■■■■■

ENDOCRINE SYSTEM
■■■

CIRCULATION AND IMMUNE SYSTEM
■■■■

SKIN, MUSCLES AND BODY TISSUES
■■■■■

RESPIRATORY SYSTEM
■■■■■

DIGESTIVE SYSTEM
■■■

URINARY SYSTEM
■■■

REPRODUCTIVE SYSTEM
■■■■

CAUTIONS

BOTANICAL FAMILY

## PROPERTIES > USES

calming, tonic > calms excitement

hormone like > prostate

antiviral, bactericidal >

antiseptic, parasiticide > arthritis, rheumatism

decongestant, stimulant > bronchitis, pneumonia

parasiticide, tonic > liver, pancreas, parasites

decongestant > prostate

antiseptic > infections

Use with care because of the high phenol content.

Lamiaceae.

Herb: distilled flowering herb : hearty warming aroma : top note.
Ocimum gratissimum eugenoliferum is a distinct oil from ocimum gratissimum thymo-liferum with eugenol as its main phenol content. Maximum oil quantities are obtained during mass blooming time. The eugenol content drops by 10% two days after harvesting.

Chemical constituents may include:

■ cadinene
■ a-pinene, b-pinene, ocimene

■ a-terpinol, linalool
■ eugenol, methyl chavicol (estragole)

# BASIL EXOTIC REUNION
### Ocimum basilicum

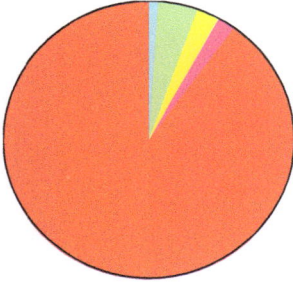

| | | |
|---|---|---|
| 🟦 | esters | yes |
| 🟦 | ketones | 1.0% |
| 🟩 | sesquiterpenes | yes |
| 🟩 | remainder | 4.5% |
| 🟨 | oxides | 2.5% |
| 🟧 | monoterpenes | yes |
| 🟪 | alcohols | 2.0% |
| 🟧 | phenols, phe. ethers | 90.0% |

## BODY SYSTEMS

**NERVOUS SYSTEM**

**ENDOCRINE SYSTEM**

**CIRCULATION AND IMMUNE SYSTEM**

**SKIN, MUSCLES AND BODY TISSUES**

**RESPIRATORY SYSTEM**

**DIGESTIVE SYSTEM**

**URINARY SYSTEM**

**REPRODUCTIVE SYSTEM**

CAUTIONS

BOTANICAL FAMILY

## PROPERTIES > USES

slightly antispasmodic > anxiety, balances sympathetic nervous system, depression

hormone like > prostate

antiviral, slightly bactericidal, decongestant > pulmonary artery, yellow fever, veins

antiinflammatory, antiseptic > plaques, polio, rheumatoid arthritis, tropical infections

antiviral, slightly bactericidal > bronchitis, pneumonia

antiinflammatory > gastritis, liver, pancreas

decongestant > prostate

Use with care because of the high (85%) methyl chavicol content. Avoid in pregnancy.

Lamiaceae.

Herb: distilled flowering herb : sweet herby with camphor tones aroma : top note. Although botanically classified the same as French or European Basil it is a larger plant with stronger odour and different constituents. Some practitioners discourage its use in aromatherapy.

Chemical constituents may include:

🟦 fenchyl acetate, linalyl acetate
🟦 octanone, camphor
🟨 1.8-cineole, trans-ocimene oxide

🟧 a-pinene, b-pinene
🟪 terpinen-4-ol, a-terpinol, linalool, fenchol, citronellol
🟧 methyl chavicol (estragole), eugenol, trans-anethole, methyl eugenol

5

# BASIL SWEET EUROPEAN
## Ocimum basilicum

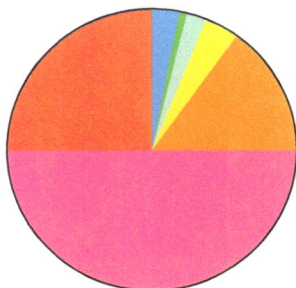

| | | |
|---|---|---|
| 🟦 | esters | 3.0% |
| 🟩 | sesquiterpenes | 1.0% |
| 🟦 | remainder | 2.0% |
| 🟨 | oxides | 4.0% |
| 🟧 | monoterpenes | 15.0% |
| 🟪 | alcohols | 50.0% |
| 🟥 | phenols, phe. ethers | 25.0% |

## BODY SYSTEMS

**NERVOUS SYSTEM**
🟦🟨🟨🟪🟧

**ENDOCRINE SYSTEM**
🟪🟧

**CIRCULATION AND IMMUNE SYSTEM**
🟦🟨🟨🟪🟧

**SKIN, MUSCLES AND BODY TISSUES**
🟦🟨🟨🟪🟧

**RESPIRATORY SYSTEM**
🟦🟨🟨🟪🟧

**DIGESTIVE SYSTEM**
🟦🟨🟨🟪🟧

**URINARY SYSTEM**
🟦🟨🟨🟪🟧

**REPRODUCTIVE SYSTEM**
🟨🟨🟪🟧

## CAUTIONS

## BOTANICAL FAMILY

## PROPERTIES > USES

antispasmodic, aphrodisiac, stimulant, tonic > anxiety, clears mind, convalescence, depression, epilepsy, migraine

hormone like, oestrogen like, temperature reducing, stimulates sweating > adrenal cortex, digestive secretions, milk production

antiviral, bactericidal, lowers blood pressure, stimulant

antifungal, antiseptic, possible irritant > acne, helps with allergies, gout, reduces uric acid, wasp stings

expectorant > catarrh, emphysema, flu, hiccoughs, restores sense of smell, sinusitis, whooping cough

stimulant > dyspepsia, flatulence, gastritis, hepatitis, liver, spasms, travel sickness, threadworms, ulcers

bactericidal > cleanses kidneys, congested prostate, cystitis

emmenagogue, stimulant > congested uterus, expels afterbirth

Safe oil provided the methyl chavicol content is low. Avoid in pregnancy.

Lamiaceae.

Herb: distilled flowering herb : clear spicy sweet aroma : top note.
Used extensively in Ayurvedic medicine. Chinese use it for epilepsy.
Chemical constituents may include:

🟦 linalyl acetate, fenchyl acetate, methyl cinnamate

🟩 b-caryophellene

🟨 1.8-cineole

🟧 a-pinene, b-pinene, g-terpinene, limonene, ocimene, p-cymene, camphene

🟪 terpinen-4-ol, a-terpineol, linalool, citronellol, geraniol

🟥 eugenol, methyl chavicol (estragole), methyl eugenol

# BASIL THYMOL
## Ocimum gratissimum thymoliferum

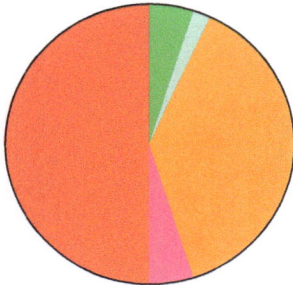

| | | |
|---|---|---|
| ■ | sesquiterpenes | 5.0% |
| ■ | remainder | 2.0% |
| ■ | acids | yes |
| ■ | monoterpenes | 38.0% |
| ■ | alcohols | 5.0% |
| ■ | phenols, phe. ethers | 50.0% |

## BODY SYSTEMS

**NERVOUS SYSTEM**
■ ■ ■

**ENDOCRINE SYSTEM**

**CIRCULATION AND IMMUNE SYSTEM**
■ ■ ■ ■

**SKIN, MUSCLES AND BODY TISSUES**
■ ■

**RESPIRATORY SYSTEM**
■ ■ ■ ■

**DIGESTIVE SYSTEM**
■ ■ ■

**URINARY SYSTEM**
■ ■ ■ ■

**REPRODUCTIVE SYSTEM**

CAUTIONS

BOTANICAL FAMILY

## PROPERTIES > USES

tonic >

antiviral, bactericidal, stimulant > balances immune system
antifungal, parasiticide >

bactericidal > bronchitis, pneumonia

antiviral > enteritis

bactericidal > excellent for cystitis

Use with care. Avoid in pregnancy.

Lamiaceae.

Herb: distilled flowering herb : herby warming aroma : top note.
Ocimum gratissimum thymoliferum is a distinct oil from ocimum gratissimum eugenoliferum with thymol as its main phenol content.

Chemical constituents may include:

■ b-caryophyllene, a-humulene, b-selinene
■ a-thujene, a-pinene, b-pinene, myrcene terpinenes, p-cymene

■ terpinen-4-ol, a-terpineol
■ thymol, carvacrol, eugenol, eugenol methyl ether, thymol methyl ether

# BENZOIN
## Styrax benzoin

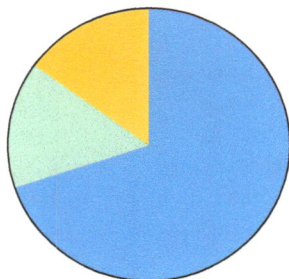

| | | |
|---|---|---|
| esters | | 70.0% |
| remainder | | 15.0% |
| acids | | 15.0% |
| aromatic aldehydes | | yes |

## BODY SYSTEMS

**NERVOUS SYSTEM**

**ENDOCRINE SYSTEM**

**CIRCULATION AND IMMUNE SYSTEM**

**SKIN, MUSCLES AND BODY TISSUES**

**RESPIRATORY SYSTEM**

**DIGESTIVE SYSTEM**

**URINARY SYSTEM**

**REPRODUCTIVE SYSTEM**

## PROPERTIES > USES

cheering, uplifting > comforting, clears mind, depression, loneliness, sadness

stimulates secretions > balances blood sugar, pancreas

astringent, tonic > cardiac, warms circulation

antioxidant, antiseptic, deodorant > arthritis, dry cracked skin, eczema, itching, rheumatism, psoriasis, ulcers, wounds

expectorant, decongestant, mucolytic > catarrh

calming > diabetes, flatulence

diuretic > cystitis

antiseptic, mucolytic > leucorrhoea

## BOTANICAL FAMILY

Styracaceae.

Tree: gum solvent : vanilla like aroma : base note.
The sap is extracted and resin is solvent extracted – strictly speaking not an essential oil. It was used in ancient times to fend off evil spirits. Used in fumigations and in incense. It is an ingredient of Friar's Balsam.

Chemical constituents may include:

coniferyl benzoate, coniferyl cinnamate
benzoic acid, cinnamic acid

benzaldehyde, vanillin

8

# BERGAMOT
## Citrus bergamia

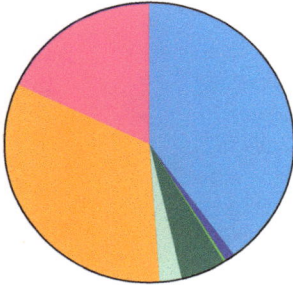

| | | |
|---|---|---|
| esters | 40.0% |
| aliphatic aldehydes | 1.0% |
| sesquiterpenes | 0.5% |
| lactones and coumarins | 5.0% |
| remainder | 2.5% |
| acids | yes |
| monoterpenes | 33.0% |
| alcohols | 18.0% |

## BODY SYSTEMS

**NERVOUS SYSTEM**

**ENDOCRINE SYSTEM**

**CIRCULATION AND IMMUNE SYSTEM**

**SKIN, MUSCLES AND BODY TISSUES**

**RESPIRATORY SYSTEM**

**DIGESTIVE SYSTEM**

**URINARY SYSTEM**

**REPRODUCTIVE SYSTEM**

CAUTIONS

BOTANICAL FAMILY

## PROPERTIES > USES

antispasmodic, calming > excellent for agitation, often first choice in cases of depression
stimulates secretions > bile

antiviral, bactericidal >

antifungal, antiseptic, phototoxic > boils, chicken pox, cold sores, herpes, pruritus, psoriasis, shingles
antiviral > colds, flu, tonsillitis

stimulates secretions > gall stones, indigestion, internal parasites
antiseptic > cystitis

antifungal, antiseptic > leucorrhoea, thrush

Use with care, skin may be photosensitive after application.

Rutaceae: this family generally aids digestion and skin problems.

Tree: cold expression peel of nearly ripe fruit : light citrus aroma : top note.
Has gentle action covering a wide range of therapeutic uses. Used in Earl Grey tea.

Chemical constituents may include:

linalyl acetate
citral
b-bisabolene

bergaptene
b-pinene, g-terpinene, a-terpinene, limonene
linalool, geraniol

# BLACK PEPPER
## Piper nigrum

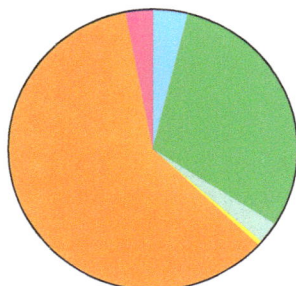

| | | |
|---|---|---|
| ☐ | ketones | 4.0% |
| ☐ | sesquiterpenes | 30.6% |
| ☐ | remainder | 2.3% |
| ☐ | oxides | yes |
| ☐ | acids | yes |
| ☐ | aromatic aldehydes | 0.1% |
| ☐ | monoterpenes | 60.0% |
| ☐ | alcohols | 3.0% |
| ☐ | phenols, phe. ethers | yes |

## BODY SYSTEMS

### PROPERTIES > USES

NERVOUS SYSTEM

analgesic, aphrodisiac, antispasmodic, tonic >
neuralgia, Raynaud's disease
lowers fever, temperature control >

ENDOCRINE SYSTEM

CIRCULATION AND IMMUNE SYSTEM

antiviral, bactericidal, decongestant, stimulant >
anaemia, angina, cardiac

SKIN, MUSCLES AND BODY TISSUES

antiseptic > aches and pains, bruises, chilblains,
rhuematism, rhuematoid arthritis, toothache,
temporary paralysis

RESPIRATORY SYSTEM

expectorant, decongestant > bronchitis, catarrh

DIGESTIVE SYSTEM

stimulant > constipation, flatulence, indigestion,
liver, pancreas, reduces fat, tones colon muscles

URINARY SYSTEM

diuretic >

REPRODUCTIVE SYSTEM

stimulant > frigidity

## CAUTIONS

Use with care, too much may overstimulate the
kidneys.

## BOTANICAL FAMILY

Piperaceae.

Shrub: distilled fruits : sharp spicy aroma : middle note.
Used for over 4000 years in India particularly for urinary and liver disorders.

Chemical constituents may include:
- ☐ piperitone, dihydrocarvone
- ☐ b-caryophyllene, bisabolene
- ☐ caryophyllene oxide, 1.8-cineole
- ☐ piperonal
- ☐ limonene, a-pinene, b-pinene, sabinene, terpinenes, phellandrene, myrcene, camphene, thujene
- ☐ terpinen-4-ol, a-terpineol, linalool
- ☐ myristicin, safrole

# CADE
## Juniperus oxycedrus

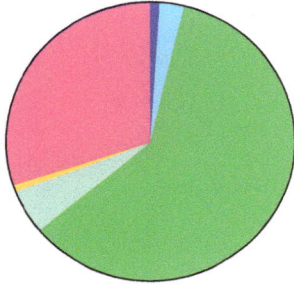

| | | |
|---|---|---|
| ■ | esters | yes |
| ■ | aliphatic aldehydes | 1.0% |
| ■ | ketones | 3.0% |
| ■ | sesquiterpenes | 60.0% |
| ■ | remainder | 5.3% |
| ■ | acids | 0.7% |
| ■ | alcohols | 30.0% |
| ■ | phenols, phe. ethers | yes |

## BODY SYSTEMS

**NERVOUS SYSTEM**
■ ■ ■ ■ ■

**ENDOCRINE SYSTEM**

**CIRCULATION AND IMMUNE SYSTEM**

**SKIN, MUSCLES AND BODY TISSUES**
■ ■ ■ ■ ■ ■ ■

**RESPIRATORY SYSTEM**

**DIGESTIVE SYSTEM**
■ ■

**URINARY SYSTEM**

**REPRODUCTIVE SYSTEM**

CAUTIONS

BOTANICAL FAMILY

## PROPERTIES > USES

analgesic, calming > anxiety

antiinflammatory, antiseptic, parasiticide, possible irritant > cuts, dandruff, dermititis, eczema, spots

parasiticide > worms

Use with care when treating inflammatory conditions or allergic skin conditions.

Cupressaceae: this family generally aids nervous tension, rheumatism and cellulite.

Tree: distilled wood : leathery aroma : base note.
Used extensively in dermatological creams and ointments as well as in veterinary medicine. Historically used for cutaneous and chronic skin problems.

Chemical constituents may include:

■ carvone
■ b-caryophyllene, cadinene, cedrene

■ cadinol, pseudo-cedrol
■ p-cresol, guaiacol

# CARAWAY SEED
## Carum carvi

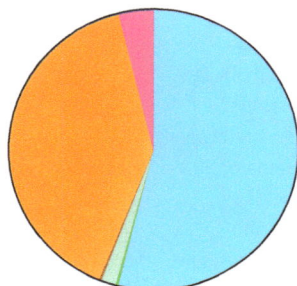

| | | |
|---|---|---|
| ketones | | 54.0% |
| sesquiterpenes | | 0.1% |
| lactones and coumarins | | yes |
| remainder | | 1.8% |
| acids | | yes |
| aromatic aldehydes | | 0.1% |
| monoterpenes | | 40.0% |
| alcohols | | 4.0% |

## BODY SYSTEMS

**NERVOUS SYSTEM**

**ENDOCRINE SYSTEM**

**CIRCULATION AND IMMUNE SYSTEM**

**SKIN, MUSCLES AND BODY TISSUES**

**RESPIRATORY SYSTEM**

**DIGESTIVE SYSTEM**

**URINARY SYSTEM**

**REPRODUCTIVE SYSTEM**

CAUTIONS

BOTANICAL FAMILY

## PROPERTIES > USES

antispasmodic, tonic > anger, vertigo

hormone like, tonic > stimulates milk production and bile production

stimulant, bactericidal > blood purifier, immune stimulant, possible aid for cancer (2)

antifungal, antiseptic > cell regenerator, scalp problems, toothache

mucolytic > bronchitis, catarrh

stimulant > calms gastric and intestinal spasms, flatulence, indigestion, stimulates bile production

abortive > stimulates milk production

Avoid for pregnant women, babies and young children.

Umbelliferae: this family generally aids digestion.

Herb: distilled fruits, dried ripe seed : peppery sharp yet sweet aroma : top note. Used widely in cooking – it aids digestion. Also used in aperitifs.

Chemical constituents may include:
- carvone, dihydrocarvone
- caryophyllene
- cuminaldehyde
- limonene, phellandrene
- cis-carveol, dihydrocarveol

# CARROT SEED
## Daucus carota

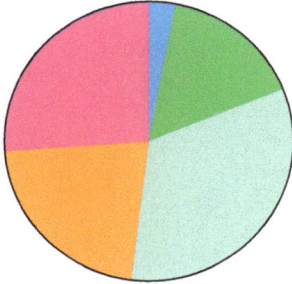

| | | |
|---|---|---|
| 🟦 | esters | 3.0% |
| 🟩 | sesquiterpenes | 16.0% |
| 🟩 | remainder | 33.0% |
| 🟨 | acids | yes |
| 🟧 | monoterpenes | 22.0% |
| 🟪 | alcohols | 26.0% |
| 🟧 | phenols, phe. ethers | yes |

## BODY SYSTEMS

**NERVOUS SYSTEM**
🟦🟩🟨🟪🟧

**ENDOCRINE SYSTEM**
🟩🟨🟪🟧

**CIRCULATION AND IMMUNE SYSTEM**
🟩🟨🟪🟧

**SKIN, MUSCLES AND BODY TISSUES**
🟦🟩🟨🟪🟧🟧

**RESPIRATORY SYSTEM**
🟩🟨🟪🟧

**DIGESTIVE SYSTEM**
🟦🟩🟨🟪🟧

**URINARY SYSTEM**
🟩🟨🟪🟧

**REPRODUCTIVE SYSTEM**
🟦🟩🟨🟪🟧

## BOTANICAL FAMILY

## PROPERTIES > USES

calming, tonic > anxiety

hormone like, tonic to hormone production > regulates menstrual cycle, thyroid regulator

bactericidal, decongestant, lowers blood pressure > anaemia, dilates blood vessels, immune stimulant

antiaging, antiseptic, cell regenerator > chilblains, eczema, gout, psoriasis, excellent for skin care, ulcers, wounds

bactericidal > bronchitis, strengthens mucous membranes

bactericidal, calming > anorexia, diarrhoea, flatulance, hepatitis, jaundice, liver problems, ulcers

diuretic > cystitis, purifies kidneys, kidney stones

hormone like > aids conception, helps infertility

Umbelliferae: this family generally aids digestion.

Plant wild carrot: distilled seed : dry sweet aroma : middle note.
Excellent for general health and well being. Used widely in food flavouring.

Chemical constituents may include:

🟦 geranyl acetate
🟩 daucene, bisabolene, elemene, caryophyllene
🟧 limonene, a-pinene, b-pinene

🟪 carotol, daucol, linalool, geraniol
🟧 asarone

# CATNIP
## Nepata cataria

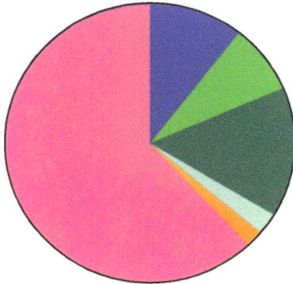

| | | |
|---|---|---|
| ☐ | esters | yes |
| ☐ | aliphatic aldehydes | 10.5% |
| ☐ | sesquiterpenes | 8.0% |
| ☐ | lactones and coumarins | 15.0% |
| ☐ | remainder | 2.5% |
| ☐ | acids | yes |
| ☐ | monoterpenes | 2.0% |
| ☐ | alcohols | 62.0% |
| ☐ | phenols, phe. ethers | yes |

## BODY SYSTEMS

NERVOUS SYSTEM

ENDOCRINE SYSTEM

CIRCULATION AND IMMUNE SYSTEM

SKIN, MUSCLES AND BODY TISSUES

RESPIRATORY SYSTEM

DIGESTIVE SYSTEM

URINARY SYSTEM

REPRODUCTIVE SYSTEM

BOTANICAL FAMILY

## PROPERTIES > USES

antispasmodic, calming, uplifting > nervous depression

strongly antiviral >

antiinflammatory, antiseptic > arthritis, herpes, rheumatism

calming > gall stones, irritable bowel syndrome

antiseptic > infections

Lamiaceae.

Herb: distilled flower tips : strong pungent aroma due to nepetalactone : top note.
Unusual essential oil in its 15% lactones This ties up with its recommendation for nervous depression.

Chemical constituents may include:
- neral, geranial
- b-caryophyllene, a-humulene
- nepetalactone, epinepetalactone, dihydronepetalactone
- myrcene, limonene, ocimene
- citronellol, geraniol

# CEDAR TEXAS
## Juniperus ashei

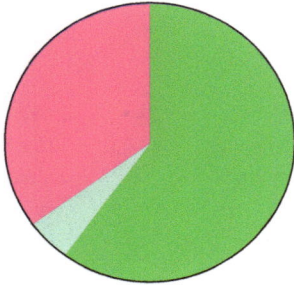

| | | |
|---|---|---|
| ■ sesquiterpenes | | 60.0% |
| □ remainder | | 5.0% |
| ■ alcohols | | 35.0% |

BODY SYSTEMS

**NERVOUS SYSTEM**
■■

**ENDOCRINE SYSTEM**

**CIRCULATION AND IMMUNE SYSTEM**
■■

**SKIN, MUSCLES AND BODY TISSUES**
■■

**RESPIRATORY SYSTEM**
■■■

**DIGESTIVE SYSTEM**

**URINARY SYSTEM**
■■

**REPRODUCTIVE SYSTEM**
■■

CAUTIONS

BOTANICAL FAMILY

PROPERTIES > USES

antispasmodic, sedative > nervous tension, stress

astringent, bactericidal, decongestant, stimulant > phlebitis

antiseptic > acne, arthritis, dandruff, eczema, greasy hair, haemorrhoids, psoriasis, rheumatism, varicose veins

expectorant > bronchitis, catarrh, coughs, sinusitis

diuretic > cystitis

antiseptic > leucorrhoea

Can irritate skin. Avoid in pregnancy.

Cupressaceae: this family generally aids nervous tension, rheumatism and cellulite.

Tree: distilled heartwood : sweet tar like aroma : base note.
Small 24 foot tree with crooked and twisted branches. It is felled for its essential oil.
Traditionally used to treat skin rashes, arthritis and rheumatism.

Chemical constituents may include:

■ cedrene, thujopsene          ■ cedrol, widdrol

# CEDAR VIRGINIAN RED
## Juniperus virginiana

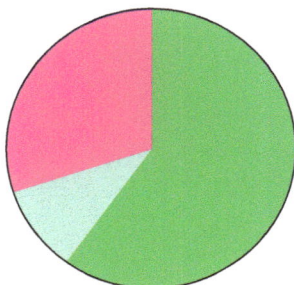

| | | |
|---|---|---|
| ■ | sesquiterpenes | 60.0% |
| ☐ | remainder | 10.0% |
| ■ | alcohols | 30.0% |

## BODY SYSTEMS

**NERVOUS SYSTEM**
■ ■

**ENDOCRINE SYSTEM**
■ ■

**CIRCULATION AND IMMUNE SYSTEM**
■ ■

**SKIN, MUSCLES AND BODY TISSUES**
■ ☐ ■

**RESPIRATORY SYSTEM**
■ ☐ ■

**DIGESTIVE SYSTEM**

**URINARY SYSTEM**
■ ■

**REPRODUCTIVE SYSTEM**
■ ■

CAUTIONS

BOTANICAL FAMILY

## PROPERTIES > USES

antispasmodic, good for meditation, sedative, tonic > nervous tension

balancing > controls sebum production, good for chronic conditions

astringent, decongestant > internal and external haemorrhoids, phlebitis, ulcers

antifungal, antiseptic, balm, insecticide > acne, baldness, chronic arthritis and rheumatism, dandruff, eczema, oily skin

expectorant > catarrh (drying effect), bronchitis

diuretic > cystitis (calms burning pain), kidney tonic

possibly abortive > leucorrhoea

Can irritate skin. Avoid in pregnancy.

Cupressaceae: this family generally aids nervous tension, rheumatism and cellulite.

Tree: distilled sawdust, previously heartwood : dry sandalwood like aroma : base note. Large redwood 100 feet, trunk diameter 5 feet. Derivation of the word cedar means spiritual strength, symbol of good faith. Used as incense and in mummification.

Chemical constituents may include:

■ cadinene, cedrene, thujopsene, cuparene

■ cedrol, cedrenol, widdrol, g-eudesmol

# CEDARWOOD ATLAS
## Cedrus atlantica

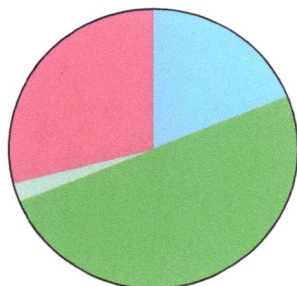

| | | |
|---|---|---|
| ☐ | ketones | 19.0% |
| ☐ | sesquiterpenes | 50.0% |
| ☐ | remainder | 2.0% |
| ☐ | alcohols | 29.0% |

## BODY SYSTEMS

**NERVOUS SYSTEM**
☐☐☐

**ENDOCRINE SYSTEM**
☐☐☐

**CIRCULATION AND IMMUNE SYSTEM**
☐☐☐

**SKIN, MUSCLES AND BODY TISSUES**
☐☐☐

**RESPIRATORY SYSTEM**
☐☐☐

**DIGESTIVE SYSTEM**

**URINARY SYSTEM**
☐☐☐

**REPRODUCTIVE SYSTEM**
☐

CAUTIONS

BOTANICAL FAMILY

## PROPERTIES > USES

aphrodisiac, sedative > neuralgia

balancing > balances sebum production

bactericidal, decongestant > clears arteries, cellulite, stimulates lympth circulation

antifungal, antiseptic > arthritis, hair loss, pruritus, rheumatism, wounds

mucolytic > bronchitis, TB

diuretic > cystitis

mucolytic > leucorrhoea

Best avoided in pregnancy.

Pinaceae: this family is highly antiseptic and generally aids respiratory problems.

Tree: distilled wood : woody dry aroma : base note.
Majestic 120 foot tree. Hardwood with strong aroma. Traditionally used for bronchial and urinary tract infections also for preservation and incense. Employed in traditional Tibetan medicine.

Chemical constituents may include:

☐ a-atlantone, g-atlantone
☐ cedrene, caryophyllene, thujopsene, cadinene

☐ atlantol, cedrol

# CHAMOMILE GERMAN
## Matricaria recutica

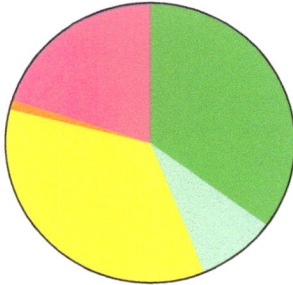

| | | |
|---|---|---|
| 🟩 | sesquiterpenes | 35.0% |
| 🟩 | lactones and coumarins | yes |
| ⬜ | remainder | 9.0% |
| 🟨 | oxides | 35.0% |
| 🟧 | monoterpenes | 1.0% |
| 🟥 | alcohols | 20.0% |

## BODY SYSTEMS

NERVOUS SYSTEM
🟩🟩⬜🟧🟥

ENDOCRINE SYSTEM
🟩🟩⬜🟧🟥

CIRCULATION AND IMMUNE SYSTEM
🟩⬜🟨🟧🟥

SKIN, MUSCLES AND BODY TISSUES
🟩🟩⬜🟨🟧🟥

RESPIRATORY SYSTEM

DIGESTIVE SYSTEM
🟩🟩⬜🟨🟥

URINARY SYSTEM
🟩⬜🟥

REPRODUCTIVE SYSTEM
🟩⬜🟨🟧🟥

BOTANICAL FAMILY

## PROPERTIES > USES

analgesic, antispasmodic > insomnia, migraine, stress

hormone like, temperature reducing, stimulates secretions > balances menstrual cycle, bile

bactericidal, decongestant > fever, stimulates production of leucocytes

antiinflammatory > acne, allergies, boils, burns, insect bites, psoriasis, rashes, rheumatism, toothache, ulcers, wounds

calming, tonic, vermifuge > calms digestion, gastric ulcers, stimulates bile production

bactericidal > cystitis

balancing > amenorrhoea, heavy periods, painful periods

Compositae: this family is generally soothing especially for skin and digestion.

Herb: distilled flower heads : warm herby aroma : middle note.
Used in traditional medicine (4) good for all states of tension and nervous reactions to stress. The deep blue colour of the oil is due to the chamazulene which forms during distillation.

Chemical constituents may include:

🟩 chamazulene, farnesene  🟥 a-bisabolol
🟨 a-bisabolol oxide  ⬜ en-yn-dicycloether, cis-spiro ether

# CHAMOMILE MAROC
## Ormenis multicaulis

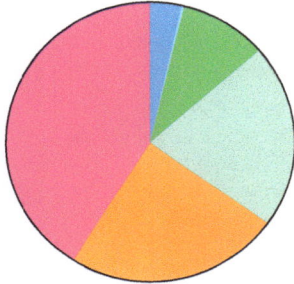

| | | |
|---|---|---|
| 🟦 | esters | 3.5% |
| 🟦 | ketones | 0.5% |
| 🟩 | sesquiterpenes | 9.7% |
| 🟩 | remainder | 21.3% |
| 🟨 | oxides | yes |
| 🟧 | monoterpenes | 24.0% |
| 🟥 | alcohols | 41.0% |
| 🟧 | phenols, phe. ethers | yes |

BODY SYSTEMS

NERVOUS SYSTEM
🟦🟦🟨🟧🟥🟧

ENDOCRINE SYSTEM
🟦🟩🟥🟧

CIRCULATION AND IMMUNE SYSTEM
🟦🟩🟨🟥🟧

SKIN, MUSCLES AND BODY TISSUES
🟦🟦🟧🟥🟧

RESPIRATORY SYSTEM

DIGESTIVE SYSTEM
🟦🟩🟨🟥🟧

URINARY SYSTEM
🟦🟩🟨🟥🟧

REPRODUCTIVE SYSTEM
🟦🟦🟩🟨🟥🟧

BOTANICAL FAMILY

PROPERTIES > USES

aphrodisiac, tonic > depression, insomnia,
irritability, headache
hormone like, stimulates secretions >

bactericidal, decongestant, general tonic >
decongestant for arteries
antiseptic, parasiticide > eczema, dry cracked skin,
infected pus

stimulates secretions > bile and gastric juices, liver
and spleen congestion, parasites
bactericidal > cystitis, prostate problems

emmenagogue > amenorrhoea, menopause, painful
periods

Compositae: this family is generally soothing
especially for the skin and digestion.

Herb: distilled flowerheads : fresh balsamic aroma : middle note.
Distantly related to the roman and german chamomiles.

Chemical constituents may include:

🟦 benzyl acetate, bornyl acetate,
   bornyl butyrate
🟦 camphor, pinocarvone
🟩 germacrene, b-caryophyllene,
   bisabolene

🟨 1.8-cineole
🟧 a-pinene, myrcene
🟥 santolina alcohol, yomogi alcohol, artemisia
   alcohol, trans-pinocarveol
🟧 eugenol

# CHAMOMILE ROMAN
## Chamaemelum nobile

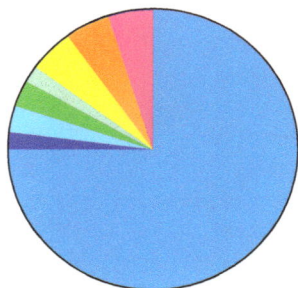

| | | |
|---|---|---|
| 🟦 | esters | 75.0% |
| 🟦 | aliphatic aldehydes | 2.0% |
| 🟦 | ketones | 3.0% |
| 🟩 | sesquiterpenes | 3.0% |
| 🟩 | lactones and coumarins | yes |
| 🟩 | remainder | 2.0% |
| 🟨 | oxides | 5.0% |
| 🟨 | acids | yes |
| 🟧 | monoterpenes | 5.0% |
| 🟥 | alcohols | 5.0% |

## BODY SYSTEMS

**NERVOUS SYSTEM**

🟦🟦🟦🟩🟧🟥

**ENDOCRINE SYSTEM**

🟦🟦🟦🟩🟩🟥

**CIRCULATION AND IMMUNE SYSTEM**

🟩🟨🟧🟥

**SKIN, MUSCLES AND BODY TISSUES**

🟦🟦🟦🟩🟩🟨🟨🟧🟥

**RESPIRATORY SYSTEM**

🟦🟦🟦🟩🟩

**DIGESTIVE SYSTEM**

🟦🟦🟦🟩🟩🟨🟧🟥

**URINARY SYSTEM**

**REPRODUCTIVE SYSTEM**

🟦🟦🟦🟩🟩🟨🟧🟥

## BOTANICAL FAMILY

## PROPERTIES > USES

antispasmodic, calming, sedative > depression, insomnia, irritability, neuralgia, neuritis, migraine, shocks
temperature reducing, causes sweating > balances menstrual cycle
bactericidal > anaemia

antiinflammatory > back pain, conjunctivitis, cracked nipples, gout, irritation, psoriasis, surgical scars
calming > nervous asthma

calming, parasiticide > intestinal colic, flatulence, jaundice, liver, stimulates appetite

emmenagogue > amenorrhoea, nervous menstrual problems, menopause, painful periods

Compositae: this family is generally soothing especially for the skin and digestion.

Herb: distilled flowerheads : fruity apple like aroma : middle note.
Highly respected for its calming influence on all systems. Known as the plant's physician as it protects neighbouring plants from infections. Potent sedative as well as long lasting antiinflammatory.

Chemical constituents may include:

🟦 angelates, tiglates, butyrates, propionates
🟦 pinocarvone
🟩 chamazulene, caryophyllene

🟨 1.8-cineole
🟧 a-pinene, sabinene
🟥 farnesol, nerolidol, a--terpineol, trans-pinocarveol

# CINNAMON LEAF
## Cinnamomum zeylanicum

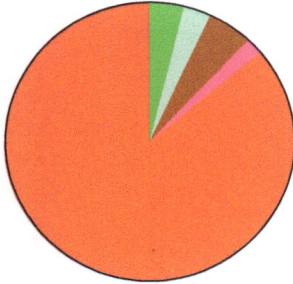

| | | |
|---|---|---|
| ■ | esters | yes |
| ■ | sesquiterpenes | 4.0% |
| ■ | remainder | 3.0% |
| ■ | aromatic aldehydes | 5.0% |
| ■ | monoterpenes | yes |
| ■ | alcohols | 2.0% |
| ■ | phenols, phe. ethers | 86.0% |

BODY SYSTEMS

NERVOUS SYSTEM
■ ■ ■ ■ ■ ■

ENDOCRINE SYSTEM
■ ■ ■ ■

CIRCULATION AND IMMUNE SYSTEM
■ ■ ■ ■ ■ ■

SKIN, MUSCLES AND BODY TISSUES
■ ■ ■ ■ ■ ■

RESPIRATORY SYSTEM
■ ■ ■ ■ ■ ■

DIGESTIVE SYSTEM
■ ■ ■ ■ ■ ■

URINARY SYSTEM

REPRODUCTIVE SYSTEM
■

CAUTIONS

BOTANICAL FAMILY

PROPERTIES > USES

antispasmodic, aphrodisiac, stimulant > neuralgia

raises body temperature, stimulates secretions >
gastric, glandular tonic, promotes menstruation,
stimulates tears and mucous

antiviral, astringent, bactericidal, heart tonic >
arrests bleeding, blood purifier

antifungal, antioxidant, antiseptic, tonic > insects,
toothache, warts

antispasmodic > eases breathing, fainting fits

stimulates secretions > anorexia, diarrhoea,
flatulence, nausea, saliva flow

emmenagogue > can help in childbirth,
leucorrhoea

Avoid in pregnancy. Powerful oil, use with care.

Lauraceae: this family is usually powerful and
stimulating.

Tree: distilled leaves : musty sweet sharp aroma : base note.
Pheonix collected cinnamon, myrrh and spikenard for the magic fire. Cinnamon was used
in love potions and incense.

Chemical constituents may include:
■ benzyl benzoate, benzyl acetate,      ■ a-pinene, p-cymene
  cinnamyl acetate                      ■ geraniol, borneol, linalool, terpineol
■ b-caryophyllene                       ■ eugenol, safrole, aceteugenol
■ cinnamaldehyde, methyl vanillin

# CLARY SAGE

## Salvia sclarea

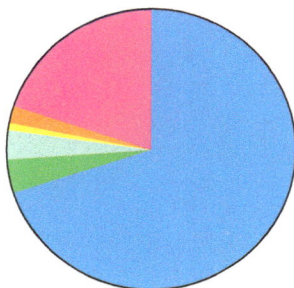

| | | |
|---|---|---|
| 🟦 | esters | 70.0% |
| 🟪 | aliphatic aldehydes | yes |
| 🟦 | ketones | yes |
| 🟩 | sesquiterpenes | 4.0% |
| 🟢 | lactones and coumarins | yes |
| ⬜ | remainder | 3.2% |
| 🟨 | oxides | 0.8% |
| 🟨 | acids | yes |
| 🟧 | monoterpenes | 2.0% |
| 🟧 | alcohols | 20.0% |
| 🟧 | phenols, phe. ethers | yes |

## BODY SYSTEMS

NERVOUS SYSTEM

🟦🟪🟦🟩🟢🟨🟧🟥🟧

ENDOCRINE SYSTEM

🟦🟦🟧

CIRCULATION AND IMMUNE SYSTEM

🟦🟪🟦🟩🟨🟥🟧

SKIN, MUSCLES AND BODY TISSUES

🟦🟪🟦🟩🟨🟥🟧

RESPIRATORY SYSTEM

🟦🟪🟦🟢

DIGESTIVE SYSTEM

🟦🟪🟦🟩🟨🟥

URINARY SYSTEM

REPRODUCTIVE SYSTEM

🟦🟪🟦🟩🟧🟥🟧

## CAUTIONS

## BOTANICAL FAMILY

## PROPERTIES > USES

antispasmodic, calming, sedative, tonic > convalescence, convulsions, panic attacks, postnatal depression
controls sebum production, oestrogen like, sweating > menopausal problems
bactericidal, decongestant, lowers blood pressure > cholesterol, phlebitis, varicose veins
antifungal, antiinflammatory, deodorant > baldness, dandruff, greasy hair, haemorrhoids, mature skin, puffy skin
calming > asthma

calming > diabetes, flatulence

uterine tonic > amenorrhoea, assists childbirth, menopausal problems, scanty periods
Avoid in cases of hormone related cancers. Avoid in pregnancy. Do not use if alcohol has been consumed.
Lamiaceae.

Herb: distilled flower stalks : nutty earthy aroma : top note.
Name comes from 'clarus' meaning clear and was used for clearing mucous from the eyes.
There are several different chemotypes, some oils are lower in esters and higher in alcohols.
Chemical constituents may include:

🟦 linalyl acetate, geranyl acetate, neryl acetate
🟪 caryophyllenal
🟦 thujone, camphor
🟩 caryophyllene, germacrene, bourbonene

🟨 1.8-cineole, caryophyllene oxide
🟧 a-pinene, b-pinene, myrcene, limonene, phellandrene
🟥 linalool, sclareol, a-terpineol, a-bisabolol
🟧 methyl hexyl ether

# CLOVE BUD
## Syzygium aromaticum

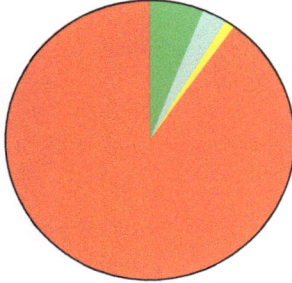

| | | |
|---|---|---|
| 🟦 | esters | yes |
| 🟩 | sesquiterpenes | 6.0% |
| 🟩 | remainder | 3.0% |
| 🟨 | oxides | 1.0% |
| 🟧 | monoterpenes | yes |
| 🟥 | phenols, phe. ethers | 90.0% |

## BODY SYSTEMS

**NERVOUS SYSTEM**
🟦🟩🟨🟧🟥

**ENDOCRINE SYSTEM**
🟩🟧🟥

**CIRCULATION AND IMMUNE SYSTEM**
🟩🟧🟥

**SKIN, MUSCLES AND BODY TISSUES**
🟦🟩🟨🟧🟥

**RESPIRATORY SYSTEM**
🟩🟨🟧🟥

**DIGESTIVE SYSTEM**
🟦🟩🟧🟥

**URINARY SYSTEM**
🟦🟩🟨🟧🟥

**REPRODUCTIVE SYSTEM**
🟦🟩🟧🟥

CAUTIONS

BOTANICAL FAMILY

## PROPERTIES > USES

analgesic, antispasmodic, stimulating > memory loss, neuralgia, polio, Raynaud's disease
hormone like > balances thyroid problems

antiviral, bactericidal, raises blood pressure > chlorosis, Hodgkin's disease
antioxidant, strong air antiseptic > clothes moths, herpes, infected acne, mosquitoes, rheumatoid arthritis, toothache, ulcers, wounds
bactericidal > bronchitis, sinusitis, TB

stimulates secretions > bowel spasm, dysentery, enteritis, liver tonic, saliva
tonic > cystitis, kidney tonic

uterine tonic > assists childbirth, frigidity, impotence, muscle toner

Check for skin irritation. Use well diluted < 1%.

Myrtaceae: this family is generally stimulating and good for the respiratory tract.

Tree: distilled buds : strong spicy aroma : base note.
Used in traditional medicine for alleviating toothache. It prevents the spread of contagious diseases such as plague. Used in many modern pharmaceuticals.

Chemical constituents may include:
🟩 b-caryophyllene, humulenes
🟨 caryophyllene oxide, humulene oxide
🟧 pinenes
🟥 eugenol, isoeugenol, aceteugenol

# CORIANDER
## Coriandrum sativum

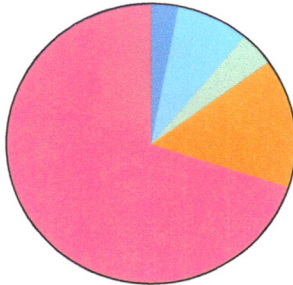

| | | |
|---|---|---|
| ■ | esters | 3.0% |
| ■ | aliphatic aldehydes | yes |
| ■ | ketones | 8.0% |
| ■ | lactones and coumarins | yes |
| ■ | remainder | 4.0% |
| ■ | acids | yes |
| ■ | monoterpenes | 15.0% |
| ■ | alcohols | 70.0% |
| ■ | phenols, phe. ethers | yes |

### BODY SYSTEMS

**NERVOUS SYSTEM**
■■■■■■■

**ENDOCRINE SYSTEM**
■■

**CIRCULATION AND IMMUNE SYSTEM**
■■■■■■

**SKIN, MUSCLES AND BODY TISSUES**
■■■■■■■■

**RESPIRATORY SYSTEM**
■■■■■

**DIGESTIVE SYSTEM**
■■■■■■■

**URINARY SYSTEM**
■■■■■■

**REPRODUCTIVE SYSTEM**
■■■■■

### PROPERTIES > USES

analgesic, antispasmodic, euphoric, uplifting, tonic > mental fatigue, sadness

hormone like, stimulates secretions > balances menstrual cycle, glandular tonic, warming

anticoagulant, antiviral, bactericidal > purifies system

antiseptic, parasiticide > osteoarthritis, rheumatism

antiviral > flu, lungs

tonic > anorexia, colic, bad breath, enteritis, indigestion

bactericidal > cystitis

stimulates secretions > irregular periods, vaginal

### BOTANICAL FAMILY

Umbelliferae: this family generally aids digestion.

Herb: distilled seeds : sweet spicy woody aroma : top note.
Used since ancient times considered the herb of happiness with aphrodisiac properties. It is used in Benedictene and Chatreuse liqueurs.

Chemical constituents may include:
- ■ geranyl acetate, linalyl acetate
- ■ decyl aldehyde
- ■ camphor, carvone
- ■ umbelliferone, bergaptene
- ■ g-terpinene, p-cymene, a-pinene, limonene
- ■ linalool, a-terpineol, geraniol, borneol
- ■ anethole

# CYPRESS
## Cupressus sempervirens

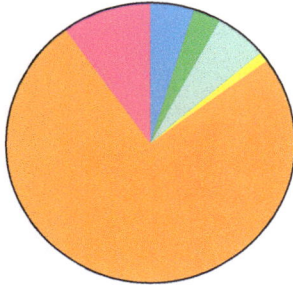

| | | |
|---|---|---|
| ■ | esters | 5.0% |
| ■ | sesquiterpenes | 3.0% |
| □ | remainder | 6.0% |
| □ | oxides | 1.0% |
| □ | acids | yes |
| ■ | monoterpenes | 75.0% |
| ■ | alcohols | 10.0% |

## BODY SYSTEMS

**NERVOUS SYSTEM**
■ ■ □ □ ■

**ENDOCRINE SYSTEM**
■ ■ □ ■

**CIRCULATION AND IMMUNE SYSTEM**
■ □ □ ■

**SKIN, MUSCLES AND BODY TISSUES**
■ ■ □ □ □ ■ ■

**RESPIRATORY SYSTEM**
■ ■ □ □ ■ ■

**DIGESTIVE SYSTEM**
□ □ ■

**URINARY SYSTEM**
□ □ ■

**REPRODUCTIVE SYSTEM**
■ ■ ■

## BOTANICAL FAMILY

## PROPERTIES > USES

antispasmodic, balances sympathetic nerve system, tonic > irritability

balancing, reduces sweating > regulates ovarian function, combats excesses

astringent, bactericidal, decongestant > constricts blood vessels

antiseptic, insecticide > broken capillaries, cellulite, haemorrhoids, pyorrhoea, rheumatism, sweaty feet

bactericidal > bronchitis, lungs, pleurisy, TB, whooping cough

stimulates secretions > liver, pancreas

decongestant, diuretic > prostate problems

balancing > irregular periods, menopause, pmt

Cupressaceae: this family generally aids nervous tension, rheumatism and cellulite.

Tree: distilled needles and twigs : clear woody spicy aroma : base note.
The island of Cyprus was named after this tree. The tree was worshipped and statues of the gods carved out of it. Sempervirens means lives for ever.

Chemical constituents may include:
■ a-terpinyl acetate, terpinen-4-yl acetate
■ cedrene, cadinene
□ 1.8-cineole, manoyl oxide

■ a-pinene, b-pinene, carene, p-cymene, camphene, limonene
■ cedrol, a-terpineol, borneol, sabinol, manool

# DILL
## Anethum graveolens

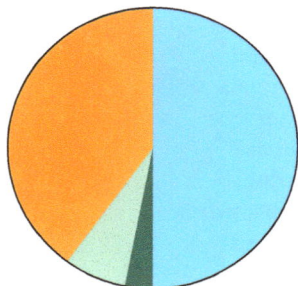

| | | |
|---|---|---|
| ketones | 50.0% |
| lactones and coumarins | 3.0% |
| remainder | 7.0% |
| monoterpenes | 40.0% |
| phenols, phe. ethers | yes |

## BODY SYSTEMS

## PROPERTIES > USES

NERVOUS SYSTEM

antispasmodic, sedative > crisis, headaches, shock

ENDOCRINE SYSTEM

increases sweating, stimulates milk production, stimulates secretions >

CIRCULATION AND IMMUNE SYSTEM

anticoagulant, bactericidal > arteries

SKIN, MUSCLES AND BODY TISSUES

antifungal, antiseptic > wounds

RESPIRATORY SYSTEM

mucolytic > bronchitis, catarrh, fevers

DIGESTIVE SYSTEM

stimulates secretions > bile, flatulence, indigestion

URINARY SYSTEM

REPRODUCTIVE SYSTEM

stimulant > assists childbirth, stimulates milk production

CAUTIONS

Avoid in pregnancy. Use with care.

BOTANICAL FAMILY

Umbelliferae: this family generally aids digestion.

Herb: distilled Indian seeds : grasslike spicy aroma : top note.
Historically used as a charm against witchcraft. Icelandic word dilla means soothing child.
There are several different chemotypes.

Chemical constituents may include:

carvone, dihydrocarvone          limonene, phellandrene, cymene, terpinene
umbelliferone, umbelliprenin

# EUCALYPTUS BLUE GUM
## Eucalyptus globulus

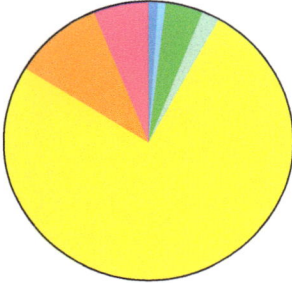

| | | |
|---|---|---|
| 🟦 | esters | 1.0% |
| 🟪 | aliphatic aldehydes | yes |
| 🟦 | ketones | 1.0% |
| 🟩 | sesquiterpenes | 4.0% |
| 🟩 | remainder | 2.0% |
| 🟨 | oxides | 76.0% |
| 🟨 | acids | yes |
| 🟧 | monoterpenes | 10.0% |
| 🟥 | alcohols | 6.0% |

## BODY SYSTEMS

**NERVOUS SYSTEM**

**ENDOCRINE SYSTEM**

**CIRCULATION AND IMMUNE SYSTEM**

**SKIN, MUSCLES AND BODY TISSUES**

**RESPIRATORY SYSTEM**

**DIGESTIVE SYSTEM**

**URINARY SYSTEM**

**REPRODUCTIVE SYSTEM**

**BOTANICAL FAMILY**

## PROPERTIES > USES

stimulant > clears head, cools emotions, migraine

stimulates secretions, temperature reducing > colds, lowers blood sugar, gall bladder, pancreas

antiviral, decongestant > malaria, reduces haemorrhage, typhoid

antiseptic > arthritis, athlete's foot, chicken pox, gnats, herpes, measles, mosquitoes

decongestant, expectorant, mucolytic > asthma, catarrh, diphtheria, laryngitis, pneumonia, scarlet fever, tonsillitis

stimulates secretions > diabetes, gall stones, pancreas

antiseptic > cystitis, nephritis

antiseptic > candida, gonorrhoea, leucorrhoea

Myrtaceae: this family is generally stimulating and good for the respiratory system.

Tree: distilled leaves and twigs : harsh camphor like aroma : top note.
An excellent oil for coughs, colds and flu.

Chemical constituents may include:
- 🟦 a-terpinyl acetate
- 🟦 pinocarvone
- 🟩 aromadendrene
- 🟨 1.8-cineole, a-pinene epoxide
- 🟧 a-pinene, limonene, p-cymene, phellandrene
- 🟥 globulol, trans-pinocarveol

# EUCALYPTUS DIVES

## Eucalyptus dives

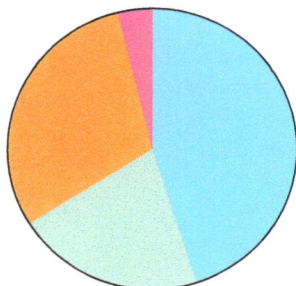

| | | |
|---|---|---|
| ■ | aliphatic aldehydes | yes |
| ■ | ketones | 45.0% |
| ■ | sesquiterpenes | yes |
| □ | remainder | 21.0% |
| □ | acids | yes |
| ■ | monoterpenes | 30.0% |
| ■ | alcohols | 4.0% |

## BODY SYSTEMS

**NERVOUS SYSTEM**
■ □ ■ ■

**ENDOCRINE SYSTEM**
■ □

**CIRCULATION AND IMMUNE SYSTEM**
□

**SKIN, MUSCLES AND BODY TISSUES**
■ □ ■ ■

**RESPIRATORY SYSTEM**
■ □ ■ ■

**DIGESTIVE SYSTEM**
□ ■

**URINARY SYSTEM**
□ ■

**REPRODUCTIVE SYSTEM**
□

CAUTIONS

BOTANICAL FAMILY

## PROPERTIES > USES

calming, sedative > exhaustion, headaches, nervous
sciatica, neuralgia

temperature reducing >

anticoagulant >

antiseptic > arthritis, cuts, rheumatism, sores, ulcers

expectorant, decongestant, mucolytic > asthma,
bronchitis, catarrh, sinusitis

stimulates secretions > gastric, aids liver function

diuretic > kidney diseases, kidney tonic

abortive > leucorrhoea

Avoid in pregnancy, and babies and young children.

Myrtaceae: this family is generally stimulating and
good for the respiratory system.

Tree: distilled leaves and twigs : camphor like spicy minty aroma : top note.
Aborigines burnt the leaves believing that the heat left the sick man and went into the fire.

Chemical constituents may include:

□ piperitone
■ b-caryophyllene

□ a-phellandrene, camphene, p-cymene, terpinene,
thujene
■ terpinen-4-ol, a-terpineol, linalool, piperitol

# EUCALYPTUS LEMON SCENTED
## Eucalyptus citriodora

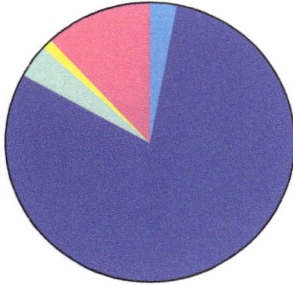

| | | |
|---|---|---|
| | esters | 3.0% |
| | aliphatic aldehydes | 80.0% |
| | ketones | yes |
| | remainder | 4.0% |
| | oxides | 1.0% |
| | monoterpenes | yes |
| | alcohols | 12.0% |

BODY SYSTEMS

NERVOUS SYSTEM

ENDOCRINE SYSTEM

CIRCULATION AND IMMUNE SYSTEM

SKIN, MUSCLES AND BODY TISSUES

RESPIRATORY SYSTEM

DIGESTIVE SYSTEM

URINARY SYSTEM

REPRODUCTIVE SYSTEM

BOTANICAL FAMILY

PROPERTIES > USES

antispasmodic, calming >

antiviral, bactericidal, lowers blood pressure > coronary, fever

antifungal, antiinflammatory, antiseptic > arthritis, chicken pox, dandruff, herpes, insects, rheumatism, scabs, sores, wounds

calming > allergies, asthma, laryngitis, sore throat

antiseptic > cystitis

stimulates secretions > excellent for candida, vaginal

Myrtaceae: this family is generally stimulating and good for the respiratory system.

Tree: distilled leaves and twigs : lemon tinged aroma : top note.
Due to its pleasant aroma it was used to perfume linen stores and to protect against silverfish and cockroaches. The synergistic action of this oil has been shown to be four times that of its component.

Chemical constituents may include:
- citronellyl butyrate, citronellyl citronellate, citronellyl acetate
- citronellal
- menthone
- 1.8-cineole
- a-pinene
- citronellol, geraniol, trans-pinocarveol

29

# EUCALYPTUS SMITHII
## Eucalyptus smithii

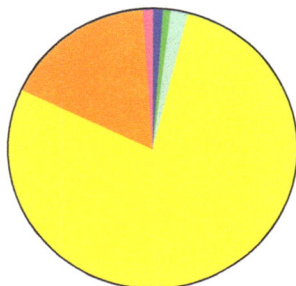

| | | |
|---|---|---|
| ☐ | esters | yes |
| ☐ | aliphatic aldehydes | 1.0% |
| ☐ | sesquiterpenes | 1.0% |
| ☐ | remainder | 2.0% |
| ☐ | oxides | 78.0% |
| ☐ | monoterpenes | 17.0% |
| ☐ | alcohols | 1.0% |
| ☐ | phenols, phe. ethers | yes |

## BODY SYSTEMS

NERVOUS SYSTEM

ENDOCRINE SYSTEM

CIRCULATION AND IMMUNE SYSTEM

SKIN, MUSCLES AND BODY TISSUES

RESPIRATORY SYSTEM

DIGESTIVE SYSTEM

URINARY SYSTEM

REPRODUCTIVE SYSTEM

BOTANICAL FAMILY

## PROPERTIES > USES

analgesic, calming (evening), stimulating (morning) > headaches

antiviral > colds, flu

antiseptic > painful joints and muscles

decongestant > asthma, bronchitis, catarrh, coughs

stimulant >

Myrtaceae: this family is generally stimulating and good for the respiratory system.

Tree: distilled leaves and twigs : penetrating aroma : top note.
Extremely high proportion of oxide gives it similar properties to eucalyptus globulus.

Chemical constituents may include:

☐ isovaleraldehyde
☐ limonene, a-pinene, p-cymene

☐ 1.8-cineole
☐ terpineol, geraniol, linalool, eudesmol

# EUCALYPTUS STAIGERIANA

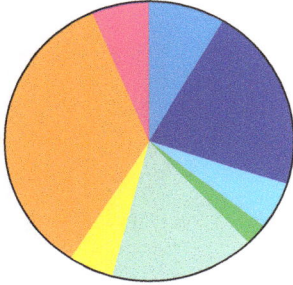

### Eucalyptus staigeriana

| | | |
|---|---|---|
| ■ | esters | 8.6% |
| ■ | aliphatic aldehydes | 21.3% |
| ■ | ketones | 5.6% |
| ■ | sesquiterpenes | 2.5% |
| ■ | remainder | 16.2% |
| ■ | oxides | 5.0% |
| ■ | monoterpenes | 34.5% |
| ■ | alcohols | 6.3% |

BODY SYSTEMS

NERVOUS SYSTEM
■ ■ ■ ■ ■

ENDOCRINE SYSTEM

CIRCULATION AND IMMUNE SYSTEM
■ ■ ■ ■

SKIN, MUSCLES AND BODY TISSUES
■ ■ ■ ■ ■ ■

RESPIRATORY SYSTEM
■ ■ ■ ■ ■ ■

DIGESTIVE SYSTEM
■ ■ ■

URINARY SYSTEM

REPRODUCTIVE SYSTEM
■ ■ ■

BOTANICAL FAMILY

PROPERTIES > USES

analgesic, calming > relaxes solar plexus

decongestant, stimulant >

antiinflammatory, antiseptic > backpain, bites, rashes, neckache, muscle cramps, sores, stings, wounds
gentle decongestant > sinusitis, sore throat

calming > digestive spasms

sexual tonic >

Myrtaceae: this family is generally stimulating and good for the respiratory system.

Tree: distilled leaves and twigs : light lemon aroma : top note.
It is likely that this eucalyptus oil is gentler than most other eucalyptus oils and might be considered for use with the elderly or young.

Chemical constituents may include:
■ menthyl acetate, geranyl acetate   ■ limonene, p-cymene
■ neral, geranial   ■ nerol, geraniol

# FENNEL SWEET
## Foeniculum vulgare

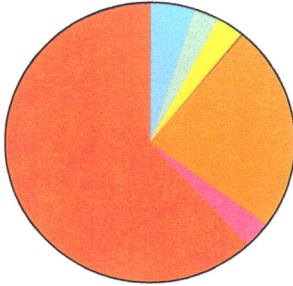

| | | |
|---|---|---|
| ☐ | ketones | 5.0% |
| ☐ | lactones and coumarins | yes |
| ☐ | remainder | 2.8% |
| ☐ | oxides | 3.0% |
| ☐ | acids | yes |
| ☐ | aromatic aldehydes | 0.2% |
| ☐ | monoterpenes | 24.0% |
| ☐ | alcohols | 3.0% |
| ☐ | phenols, phe. ethers | 62.0% |

## BODY SYSTEMS

NERVOUS SYSTEM

☐ ☐ ☐ ☐ ☐ ☐

ENDOCRINE SYSTEM

☐ ☐ ☐ ☐ ☐

CIRCULATION AND IMMUNE SYSTEM

☐ ☐ ☐ ☐ ☐

SKIN, MUSCLES AND BODY TISSUES

☐ ☐ ☐ ☐ ☐

RESPIRATORY SYSTEM

☐ ☐ ☐ ☐ ☐ ☐ ☐

DIGESTIVE SYSTEM

☐ ☐ ☐ ☐ ☐

URINARY SYSTEM

☐ ☐ ☐ ☐ ☐

REPRODUCTIVE SYSTEM

☐ ☐ ☐ ☐ ☐

CAUTIONS

BOTANICAL FAMILY

## PROPERTIES > USES

analgesic, antispasmodic, stimulant, tonic > gives strength and courage, paralysis, Raynaud's disease
hormone like, oestrogen like, increases sweating >

bactericidal, decongestant, purifies, stimulant > angina, cardiac rhythm, palpitations
antiinflammatory, antiseptic, insecticide > cellulite, dissolves boils and swellings, fluid retention, oedema, wrinkles
decongestant, tonic > asthma, bronchitis, rapid breathing, whooping cough
bactericidal > anorexia, constipation, flatulence, indigestion, parasites
diuretic > cystitis, infections, kidney stones

breast decongestant > amenorrhoea, assists childbirth, regulates menstrual cycle, stimulates milk production

Do not use with pregnant women, babies and young children. Do not use if epilepsy is suspected. Umbelliferae: this family generally aids digestion.

Herb: distilled crushed seeds : sweet aniseed like aroma : top – middle note.
Sweet fennel mimics oestrogen. Note bitter fennel comes from distilling the herb and crushed seeds and contains up to 22% ketones and is thus best avoided.

Chemical constituents may include:

☐ fenchone
☐ bergaptene, umbelliferone
☐ 1.8-cineole
☐ anisaldehyde

☐ anisic acid
☐ a-pinene, a-thujene, g-terpinene, limonene, myrcene, phellandrene
☐ fenchol
☐ trans-anethole, methyl chavicol (estragole)

# FIR NEEDLE SILVER
## Abies alba

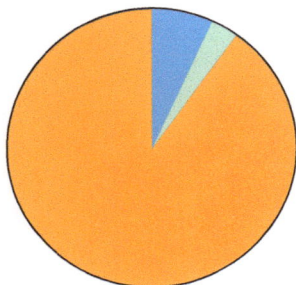

| | | |
|---|---|---|
| ⬜ | esters | 7.0% |
| 🟦 | aliphatic aldehydes | yes |
| 🟩 | sesquiterpenes | yes |
| ⬜ | remainder | 3.0% |
| 🟧 | monoterpenes | 90.0% |

BODY SYSTEMS

PROPERTIES > USES

NERVOUS SYSTEM
🟩⬜

analgesic, stimulant >

ENDOCRINE SYSTEM

CIRCULATION AND IMMUNE SYSTEM
🟩⬜

bactericidal, decongestant > arteries

SKIN, MUSCLES AND BODY TISSUES
🟦🟩🟩🟧

antiseptic > arthritis, muscular aches and pains, rheumatism

RESPIRATORY SYSTEM
🟦🟩⬜

bactericidal > bronchitis, catarrh

DIGESTIVE SYSTEM

URINARY SYSTEM

REPRODUCTIVE SYSTEM

BOTANICAL FAMILY

Pinaceae: this family is highly antiseptic and generally aids respiratory problems.

Tree: distilled needles and twigs : fragrant and soothing aroma : middle note.
It is important to know the botanical specification as there are many firs whose constituents are different.

Chemical constituents may include:
🟦 bornyl acetate
🟪 lauraldehyde, decylaldehyde

🟧 pinene, camphene, limonene

# FRANKINCENSE
## Boswellia carteri

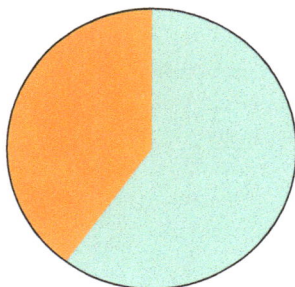

| | | |
|---|---|---|
| 🟦 | esters | yes |
| ⬜ | ketones | yes |
| 🟩 | sesquiterpenes | yes |
| 🟩 | remainder | 60.0% |
| 🟧 | monoterpenes | 40.0% |
| 🟥 | alcohols | yes |

## BODY SYSTEMS

**NERVOUS SYSTEM**
🟦⬜🟧🟥

**ENDOCRINE SYSTEM**
⬜🟩🟥

**CIRCULATION AND IMMUNE SYSTEM**
🟦⬜🟧🟥

**SKIN, MUSCLES AND BODY TISSUES**
🟦⬜🟧🟥

**RESPIRATORY SYSTEM**
🟦⬜🟧🟥

**DIGESTIVE SYSTEM**
🟦⬜🟧🟥

**URINARY SYSTEM**
🟦⬜🟧🟥

**REPRODUCTIVE SYSTEM**
🟦⬜🟧🟥

## BOTANICAL FAMILY

## PROPERTIES > USES

analgesic, antispasmodic, calming > helpful for anxious obsessional links to the past, postnatal depression

regulates secretions >

astringent, bactericidal > cancer, immune stimulant, slows breathing

antiinflammatory, antioxidant, cell regenerator > carbuncles, combats aging skin, ulcers, wounds, wrinkles

expectorant, mucolytic > asthma, bronchitis, catarrh

calming > flatulence, nephritis

bactericidal > cystitis

antiinflammatory > breast inflammation, genital infections, leucorrhoea

Buseraceae.

Tree: distilled gum resin : woody spicy aroma : base note.
Historically used as incense and aid to meditation. It was burnt to banish evil spirits from sickrooms. Considered as precious as gold in Christ's time. Chinese treated TB of lymph glands with it. Slows breathing pace. Extremely variable composition.

Chemical constituents may include:
🟦 octyl acetate
🟩 guaiene, copaene, trans-caryophyl-lene

🟧 a-pinene b-pinene, a-terpinene, diterpentene, p-cymene, thujene, myrcene, phellandrene, limonene
🟥 octanol, farnesol

# GERANIUM
## Pelargonium graveolens

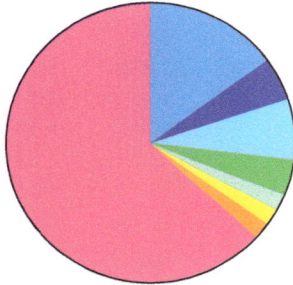

| | | |
|---|---|---|
| ■ | esters | 15.0% |
| ■ | aliphatic aldehydes | 5.0% |
| ■ | ketones | 7.0% |
| ■ | sesquiterpenes | 4.0% |
| ■ | remainder | 2.0% |
| ■ | oxides | 2.0% |
| ■ | monoterpenes | 2.0% |
| ■ | alcohols | 63.0% |

## BODY SYSTEMS

**NERVOUS SYSTEM**
■ ■ ■ ■ ■

**ENDOCRINE SYSTEM**
■ ■ ■ ■ ■

**CIRCULATION AND IMMUNE SYSTEM**
■ ■ ■ ■ ■ ■ ■

**SKIN, MUSCLES AND BODY TISSUES**
■ ■ ■ ■ ■ ■ ■

**RESPIRATORY SYSTEM**
■ ■ ■ ■ ■ ■

**DIGESTIVE SYSTEM**
■ ■ ■ ■ ■ ■ ■

**URINARY SYSTEM**
■ ■ ■ ■ ■ ■ ■

**REPRODUCTIVE SYSTEM**
■ ■ ■ ■ ■

## PROPERTIES > USES

analgesic, antispasmodic, calming > anxiety, nervous fatigue, neuralgia, Raynaud's disease

balancing, regulates hormone function > acts on the adrenal cortex

anticoagulant, bactericidal, tonic > constricts blood vessels, fluid retention, stems bleeding, varicose veins

antifungal, antiinflammatory, antioxidant, antiseptic, cell regenerator > athlete's foot, burns, haemorrhoids, impetigo, rheumatism

bactericidal > tonsillitis

decongestant, stimulant > diabetes, diarrhoea, colitis, gall bladder, jaundice, liver, pancreas

diuretic > cystitis, kidney stones

decongestant > breast congestion, candida, painful periods, pmt, uterine haemorrhage

## SUMMARY

Excellent all round balancer, eliminates waste and congestion.

## BOTANICAL FAMILY

Geraniaceae.

Plant 60cm perennial: distilled leaves and flowers : sweet rose like aroma : middle note. Traditionally a great healing plant often planted around dwellings to ward off evil spirits. Tests show strong bactericidal action.

Chemical constituents may include:

■ citronellyl formate, geranyl formate
■ citral
■ menthone
■ guaiazulene, b-caryophyllene

■ cis-rose oxide
■ phellandrene, limonene, a-pinene
■ citronellol, geraniol, linalool

# GINGER
## Zingiber officinale

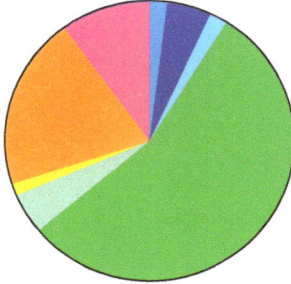

| | | |
|---|---|---|
| 🟦 | esters | 2.0% |
| 🟪 | aliphatic aldehydes | 5.0% |
| 🟦 | ketones | 2.0% |
| 🟩 | sesquiterpenes | 55.0% |
| 🟩 | remainder | 4.7% |
| 🟨 | oxides | 1.3% |
| 🟧 | monoterpenes | 20.0% |
| 🟥 | alcohols | 10.0% |

## BODY SYSTEMS

NERVOUS SYSTEM

ENDOCRINE SYSTEM

CIRCULATION AND IMMUNE SYSTEM

SKIN, MUSCLES AND BODY TISSUES

RESPIRATORY SYSTEM

DIGESTIVE SYSTEM

URINARY SYSTEM

REPRODUCTIVE SYSTEM

## PROPERTIES > USES

analgesic, antispasmodic, aphrodisiac, cheering > neuralgia

causes sweating, temperature reducing >

stimulant > angina, cholesterol, varicose veins

antioxidant, antiseptic > arthritis, back spasms, hearing, lower toothache, rheumatism, sight

expectorant > catarrh, chronic bronchitis, good for all side effects of colds

stimulant, tonic > constipation, diarrhoea, hangover, indigestion, flatulence, nausea, seasickness

balancing > disperses clots, helpful after childbirth

## BOTANICAL FAMILY

Zingiberaceae.

Herb: distilled unpeeled dried ground rhizome : warm pleasant spicy aroma : top note. Used in many ancient remedies. Prevents stomach griping when added to purgative.

Chemical constituents may include:
🟪 geranial, citronellal
🟦 gingerone
🟩 b-sesquiphellandrene, zingiberene, ar-curcumene

🟨 1.8-cineole
🟧 a-pinene, b-pinene, camphene, limonene, phellandrene
🟥 citronellol, linalool, borneol, gingerol

# GRAPEFRUIT
## Citrus paradisi

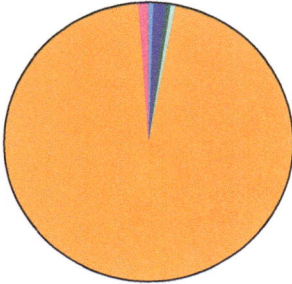

| | | |
|---|---|---|
| ⬜ | esters | 0.5% |
| 🟦 | aliphatic aldehydes | 1.0% |
| ⬜ | ketones | yes |
| 🟩 | sesquiterpenes | yes |
| 🟩 | lactones and coumarins | 0.5% |
| ⬜ | remainder | 0.5% |
| 🟧 | monoterpenes | 96.0% |
| 🟥 | alcohols | 1.0% |

## BODY SYSTEMS

**NERVOUS SYSTEM**
🟦🟦🟩🟩🟥

**ENDOCRINE SYSTEM**
⬜🟧

**CIRCULATION AND IMMUNE SYSTEM**
🟦🟧🟥

**SKIN, MUSCLES AND BODY TISSUES**
🟦🟦🟩🟩🟧🟥

**RESPIRATORY SYSTEM**

**DIGESTIVE SYSTEM**
⬜🟧

**URINARY SYSTEM**
🟦🟧🟥

**REPRODUCTIVE SYSTEM**

NOTE

BOTANICAL FAMILY

## PROPERTIES > USES

calming > relieves stress headaches and migraine

secretions > gall and liver

antiviral > colds and flu

air antiseptic > local infections, treats congested skin

secretions > breaks up gall stones, liver problems

diuretic >

Unlike other citrus oils grapefruit oil is not phototoxic.

Rutaceae: this family generally aids digestion and skin.

Tree: expressed from peel of fruit : sharp refreshing aroma : top note.
Used widely in foods and cosmetics. It is liable to oxidise quickly.

Chemical constituents may include:

🟦 geranyl acetate
🟦 citronellal, citral, sinensal
🟩 cadinene

🟩 auraptene, limettin
🟧 limonene
🟥 paradisiol, geraniol

# HYSSOP
## Hyssopus officinalis

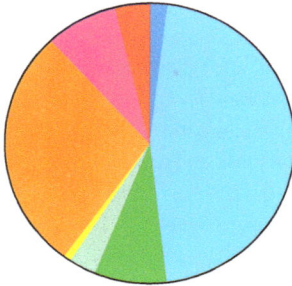

| | | |
|---|---|---|
| | esters | 2.0% |
| | ketones | 46.0% |
| | sesquiterpenes | 8.0% |
| | remainder | 3.2% |
| | oxides | 0.8% |
| | acids | yes |
| | monoterpenes | 28.0% |
| | alcohols | 8.0% |
| | phenols, phe. ethers | 4.0% |

BODY SYSTEMS

NERVOUS SYSTEM

ENDOCRINE SYSTEM

CIRCULATION AND IMMUNE SYSTEM

SKIN, MUSCLES AND BODY TISSUES

RESPIRATORY SYSTEM

DIGESTIVE SYSTEM

URINARY SYSTEM

REPRODUCTIVE SYSTEM

CAUTIONS

BOTANICAL FAMILY

PROPERTIES > USES

antispasmodic, sedative > clears head, grief, multiple sclerosis, releases emotional pain
stimulates sweating > stimulates menstrual flow

astringent, bactericidal, decongestant, regulates blood pressure > cardiac
antiinflammatory, antiseptic > bruises, dissolves boils and swellings, rheumatism, rhinopharyngitis, sinusitis
expectorant > asthma, bronchitis, catarrh, colds, chest infections, coughs, emphysema, hayfever
tonic > digestion heavy fats, flatulence, indigestion, intestinal parasites
diuretic > cystitis, kidney stones

emmenagogue > leucorrhoea

Avoid in cases of pregnancy and epilepsy.

Lamiaceae.

Herb: distilled flowering tops and leaves : warm herby penetrating aroma : middle note. Historically renowned for its cleansing properties possible help for cancer.

Chemical constituents may include:

bornyl acetate, methyl myrtenate
pinocamphone, isopinocamphone, camphor
caryophyllene, cadinene
1.8-cineole, caryophyllene oxide
b-pinene, camphene, limonene, myrcene, cis-ocimene
borneol, geraniol, linalool
methyl chavicol (estragole)

# JASMIN
## Jasminum officinale

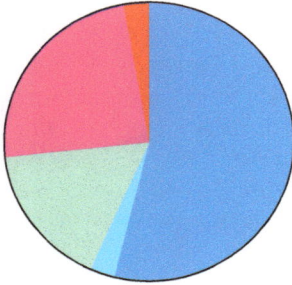

| | | |
|---|---|---|
| ■ | esters | 54.0% |
| □ | ketones | 2.7% |
| ■ | remainder | 16.6% |
| ■ | acids | yes |
| ■ | aromatic aldehydes | yes |
| ■ | alcohols | 24.0% |
| ■ | phenols, phe. ethers | 2.7% |

## BODY SYSTEMS

**NERVOUS SYSTEM**
■ ■ ■ ■ ■

**ENDOCRINE SYSTEM**
■ ■ ■

**CIRCULATION AND IMMUNE SYSTEM**

**SKIN, MUSCLES AND BODY TISSUES**
■ ■ ■ ■ ■ ■

**RESPIRATORY SYSTEM**
■ ■ ■ ■

**DIGESTIVE SYSTEM**

**URINARY SYSTEM**

**REPRODUCTIVE SYSTEM**
■ ■ ■ ■

## CAUTIONS

## BOTANICAL FAMILY

## PROPERTIES > USES

antispasmodic, aphrodisiac, calming, sedative > depression, restores confidence and thus energises
hormone like > stimulates milk production, stimulates uterine muscles in childbirth, useful after childbirth

antiseptic > good skin balm, relaxes muscles, stretch marks
antispasmodic > calms coughs, regulates and deepens breathing, relieves bronchial spasms

uterine tonic > hastens birth delivery, increases milk supply, increases sperm count, vaginal infections

Do not use during pregnancy.

Oleaceae.

Shrub: solvent extraction from flowers : exotic flowery heady aroma : base note. Considered to be the 'king' of flower oils long used in love potions.

Chemical constituents may include:

■ benzyl acetate, linalyl acetate, benzyl benzoate, methyl jasmonate, methyl anthranilate
■ cis-jasmone
■ indole
■ phenylacetic acid
■ linalool, nerol, geraniol, benzyl alcohol, farnesol, terpineol, phytols
■ eugenol

# JUNIPER BERRY
## Juniperus communis

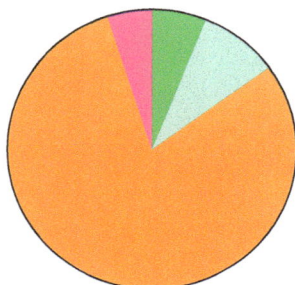

| | | |
|---|---|---|
| 🟦 | esters | yes |
| 🟩 | sesquiterpenes | 6.0% |
| 🟩 | lactones and coumarins | yes |
| ⬜ | remainder | 9.0% |
| 🟨 | oxides | yes |
| 🟨 | acids | yes |
| 🟧 | monoterpenes | 80.0% |
| 🟪 | alcohols | 5.0% |

## BODY SYSTEMS

**NERVOUS SYSTEM**
🟦🟩🟩🟧🟪

**ENDOCRINE SYSTEM**
🟩🟧🟪

**CIRCULATION AND IMMUNE SYSTEM**
🟩🟧🟪

**SKIN, MUSCLES AND BODY TISSUES**
🟦🟩🟩🟨🟨🟧🟪

**RESPIRATORY SYSTEM**

**DIGESTIVE SYSTEM**
🟦🟩🟩🟨🟧🟪

**URINARY SYSTEM**
🟩🟩🟨🟧🟪

**REPRODUCTIVE SYSTEM**
🟩🟧🟪

## CAUTIONS

## BOTANICAL FAMILY

## PROPERTIES > USES

analgesic, antispasmodic, aphrodisiac > insomnia, sciatica

causes sweating, controls sebum production, regulates menstrual cycle, stimulates secretions > antiseptic >

antiseptic > cellulite, fluid retention, eliminates uric acid, obesity, oedema, painful joints, psoriasis, stiffness

stimulates secretions > cirrhosis, clears mucous from intestines, diabetes, liver, pancreas, stimulates appetite
diuretic > cystitis, kidney stones, prostate, strangury (unable to pass urine)
regulates > amenorrhoea, assists childbirth, menstrual

Avoid in pregnancy. Do not use if kidneys are inflamed.

Cupressaceae: this family generally aids nervous tension, rheumatism and cellulite.

Shrub: distilled berries : fresh woody aroma : middle note.
Used medicinally for urinary infections. Expels uric acid from the system and is a powerful detoxifying agent.

Chemical constituents may include:
- 🟦 bornyl acetate, terpinyl acetate
- 🟩 caryophyllene, cadinene, humulene, germacrene
- 🟩 umbelliferone
- 🟨 caryophyllene oxide
- 🟧 a-pinene, b-pinene, g-terpinene, p-cymene, limonene, sabinene, thujene, myrcene, camphene
- 🟪 terpinen-4-ol, a-terpineol

# JUNIPER TWIGS
## Juniperus communis

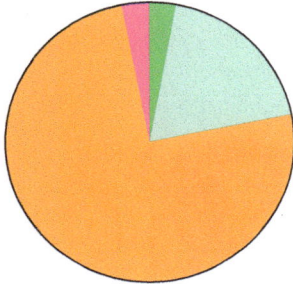

| | | |
|---|---|---|
| ■ | esters | yes |
| ■ | sesquiterpenes | 3.0% |
| ■ | lactones and coumarins | yes |
| ■ | remainder | 19.0% |
| ■ | acids | yes |
| ■ | monoterpenes | 75.0% |
| ■ | alcohols | 3.0% |

## BODY SYSTEMS

**NERVOUS SYSTEM**
■ ■ ■ ■ ■

**ENDOCRINE SYSTEM**
■

**CIRCULATION AND IMMUNE SYSTEM**
■ ■ ■

**SKIN, MUSCLES AND BODY TISSUES**
■ ■ ■ ■ ■

**RESPIRATORY SYSTEM**
■ ■ ■ ■

**DIGESTIVE SYSTEM**

**URINARY SYSTEM**
■ ■ ■ ■ ■

**REPRODUCTIVE SYSTEM**

CAUTIONS

BOTANICAL FAMILY

## PROPERTIES > USES

analgesic, antispasmodic, neurotonic > mental fatigue
reduces production of sebum >

antiseptic, decongestant > arteriosclerosis

antiinflammatory > rheumatism, fluid retention, gout, greasy hair, weeping eczema
expectorant > bronchitis, catarrh, rhinitis

diuretic > cystitis, kidney stones, prostate block, strangury (unable to pass urine)

Avoid in pregnancy. Do not use if kidneys are inflamed.

Cupressaceae: this family generally aids nervous tension, rheumatism and cellulite.

Shrub: distilled twigs : fresh terpentine like aroma : middle note.
Celtic juneprus means acrid or biting. Juniper twigs were burned to purify air in hospitals. Famous as an ingredient of gin.

Chemical constituents may include:

■ b-caryophyllene
■ a-pinene, b-pinene, g-terpinene, limonene, myrcene, sabinene, thujene

■ terpinen-4-ol

# LAVANDIN
## Lavandula hybrida

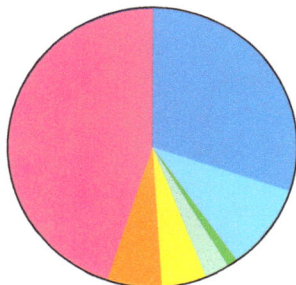

| | | |
|---|---|---|
| 🟦 | esters | 30.0% |
| 🟦 | aliphatic aldehydes | yes |
| 🟦 | ketones | 10.0% |
| 🟩 | sesquiterpenes | 1.0% |
| 🟩 | lactones and coumarins | yes |
| 🟩 | remainder | 3.0% |
| 🟨 | oxides | 5.0% |
| 🟨 | acids | yes |
| 🟫 | aromatic aldehydes | yes |
| 🟧 | monoterpenes | 6.0% |
| 🟪 | alcohols | 45.0% |
| 🟧 | phenols, phe. ethers | yes |

## BODY SYSTEMS

**NERVOUS SYSTEM**

**ENDOCRINE SYSTEM** :

**CIRCULATION AND IMMUNE SYSTEM**

**SKIN, MUSCLES AND BODY TISSUES**

**RESPIRATORY SYSTEM**

**DIGESTIVE SYSTEM**

**URINARY SYSTEM**

**REPRODUCTIVE SYSTEM**

BOTANICAL FAMILY

## PROPERTIES > USES

slightly antispasmodic, calming > anxiety, insomnia

bactericidal, lowers blood pressure, slightly decongestant, heart tonic > phlebitis
antifungal, antiinflammatory, antiseptic > allergies, cramps, dermatitis, relaxes muscles, wounds
bactericidal > colds, coughs, flu, sinusitis

Lamiaceae.

Shrub: distilled flower stalks : strong lavender aroma : middle note.
Lavandin is good for circulation and respiratory and muscle problems.

Chemical constituents may include:

🟦 linalyl acetate, bornyl acetate
🟦 camphor
🟩 caryophyllene

🟨 1.8-cineole
🟧 camphene, limonene, ocimene
🟪 linalool, a-terpineol, geraniol, lavandulol

# LAVENDER SPIKE
## Lavandula lactifolia

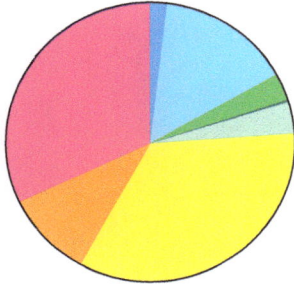

| | | |
|---|---|---|
| 🟦 | esters | 2.0% |
| 🟦 | ketones | 15.0% |
| 🟩 | sesquiterpenes | 3.0% |
| 🟩 | lactones and coumarins | 0.2% |
| 🟩 | remainder | 3.8% |
| 🟨 | oxides | 34.0% |
| 🟧 | monoterpenes | 10.0% |
| 🟥 | alcohols | 32.0% |

## BODY SYSTEMS

**NERVOUS SYSTEM**
🟦🟦🟩🟩🟨🟧🟥

**ENDOCRINE SYSTEM**
🟦🟩🟥

**CIRCULATION AND IMMUNE SYSTEM**
🟦🟦🟩🟩🟨🟧🟥

**SKIN, MUSCLES AND BODY TISSUES**
🟦🟦🟩🟩🟨🟧🟥

**RESPIRATORY SYSTEM**
🟦🟦🟩🟩🟨🟧🟥

**DIGESTIVE SYSTEM**
🟦🟦🟩🟧🟥

**URINARY SYSTEM**

**REPRODUCTIVE SYSTEM**

## PROPERTIES > USES

analgesic, antidepressant, calming > calms yet alerts, clears head, neuritis

regulating >

antiviral, bactericidal, decongestant, immune system tonic > cardiac

antifungal, antiseptic > acne, athlete's foot, bruises, midges, muscular aches and pains, rheumatism, ringworm

expectorant > bronchitis, catarrh, rhinitis

bactericidal > enteritis

BOTANICAL FAMILY        Lamiaceae.

Shrub: distilled flower stalks : fresh lavender with camphor tones aroma : middle note. More aggressive oil than true lavender due to the high camphor and cineole constituents.

Chemical constituents may include:

🟦 linalyl acetate
🟦 camphor
🟩 caryophyllene

🟨 1.8-cineole
🟧 camphene, limonene
🟥 borneol, linalool, lavandulol

# LAVENDER TRUE
## Lavandula angustifolia

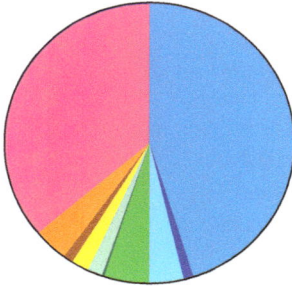

| | | |
|---|---|---|
| 🟦 | esters | 45.0% |
| 🟪 | aliphatic aldehydes | 1.0% |
| 🟦 | ketones | 4.0% |
| 🟩 | sesquiterpenes | 5.0% |
| 🟩 | lactones and coumarins | 0.3% |
| ⬜ | remainder | 1.7% |
| 🟨 | oxides | 2.0% |
| 🟫 | aromatic aldehydes | 1.0% |
| 🟧 | monoterpenes | 4.0% |
| 🟥 | alcohols | 36.0% |
| 🟧 | phenols, phe. ethers | yes |

## BODY SYSTEMS

**NERVOUS SYSTEM**

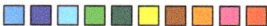

**ENDOCRINE SYSTEM**

**CIRCULATION AND IMMUNE SYSTEM**

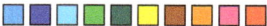

**SKIN, MUSCLES AND BODY TISSUES**

**RESPIRATORY SYSTEM**

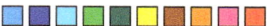

**DIGESTIVE SYSTEM**

**URINARY SYSTEM**

**REPRODUCTIVE SYSTEM**

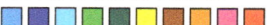

## PROPERTIES > USES

analgesic, antispasmodic, balancing, calming, cheering > anxiety, headaches, insomnia, migraines, Raynaud's disease
nervous system regulator (opposite in large doses) > stimulates menstrual cycle
antiviral, bactericidal, lowers blood pressure, mildly decongestant, heart tonic > phlebitis, varicose veins
antifungal, antiinflammatory, antiseptic, cell regenerator > arthritis, burns, radiography burns, eczema, herpes, psoriasis, spots, wounds
bactericidal > bronchitis, coughs, sinusitis, TB

stimulates, secretions > increases bile production, improves digestion heavy fats
bactericidal > cystitis

gentle emmenagogue > assists childbirth, candida, leucorrhoea, lower back massage helps expel after-birth

BOTANICAL FAMILY  Lamiaceae.

Shrub: distilled flower stalks : floral aroma : middle note. Lavere means 'to wash'. Lavender was used extensively by the Romans in their baths. Lavender oils exhibit antifungal properties.

Chemical constituents may include:
- 🟦 linalyl acetate, geranyl acetate, lavandulyl acetate
- 🟪 citral
- 🟦 octanone, camphor
- 🟩 caryophyllene
- 🟩 coumarin, umbelliferone
- 🟨 1.8-cineole, linalool oxide, caryophyllene oxide
- 🟫 cuminaldehyde, benzaldehyde
- 🟧 ocimene, camphene, limonene
- 🟥 terpinen-4-ol, a-terpineol, linalool, borneol, geraniol, lavandulol

# LEMON
## Citrus limon

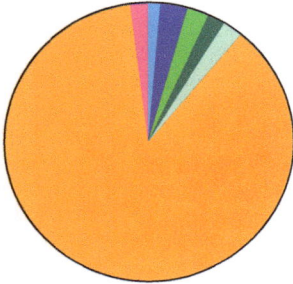

| | | |
|---|---|---|
| ■ | esters | 1.5% |
| ■ | aliphatic aldehydes | 3.0% |
| ■ | sesquiterpenes | 2.5% |
| ■ | lactones and coumarins | 2.0% |
| ■ | remainder | 2.0% |
| ■ | acids | yes |
| ■ | monoterpenes | 87.0% |
| ■ | alcohols | 2.0% |

## BODY SYSTEMS

**NERVOUS SYSTEM**
■ ■ ■ ■ ■

**ENDOCRINE SYSTEM**

**CIRCULATION AND IMMUNE SYSTEM**
■ ■ ■ ■ ■

**SKIN, MUSCLES AND BODY TISSUES**
■ ■ ■ ■ ■ ■ ■

**RESPIRATORY SYSTEM**
■ ■ ■ ■ ■ ■

**DIGESTIVE SYSTEM**
■ ■ ■ ■ ■

**URINARY SYSTEM**
■ ■

**REPRODUCTIVE SYSTEM**
■ ■ ■

## PROPERTIES > USES

antispasmodic, calming and clarifying > headaches, insomnia, nightmares

antiviral, bactericidal, lowers blood pressure, decongestant, stimulant > cellulite, cleanses, obesity, stems bleeding

antiaging, antifungal, antiseptic, skin tonic, phototoxic > arthritis, boils. brown patches, aging skin, gout, rheumatism, verrucas, warts

calming > bronchitis, catarrh

calming > diabetes, gall stones, liver, ulcers

diuretic > kidney stones

antifungal > thrush

CAUTIONS — Phototoxic.
BOTANICAL FAMILY — Rutaceae: this family generally aids digestion and skin problems.

Tree: cold expression outer fresh peel : fresh sharp aroma : top note.
General rejuvenator due to its oxidising agents. Wide therapeutic values. D-limonene has been known to dissolve gall stones.
Chemical constituents may include:

■ neryl acetate, geranyl acetate, terpinyl acetate
■ citral, citronellal, nonanal, octanal, decanal
■ b-bisabolene, a-bergamotene
■ bergaptene, bergamottin
■ limonene, a-pinene, b-pinene, g-terpinene, camphene, phellandrene, p-cymene, sabinene, myrcene
■ linalool, geraniol, octanol, a-terpineol, nonanol

# LEMONGRASS EAST INDIAN

## Cymbopogon flexuosus

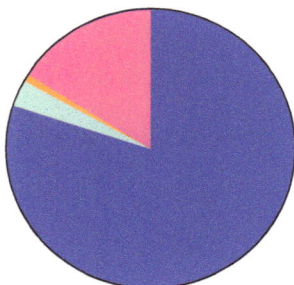

| | | |
|---|---|---|
| 🟦 | esters | yes |
| 🟪 | aliphatic aldehydes | 80.0% |
| 🟦 | ketones | yes |
| 🟩 | remainder | 3.0% |
| 🟨 | acids | yes |
| 🟧 | monoterpenes | 1.0% |
| 🟥 | alcohols | 16.0% |

BODY SYSTEMS

PROPERTIES > USES

NERVOUS SYSTEM

🟦🟪🟦🟨🟧🟥

sedative, uplifting > depression

ENDOCRINE SYSTEM

🟦🟧🟥

milk flow, reduces sweating, stimulates secretions > stimulates para-sympathetic nerves

CIRCULATION AND IMMUNE SYSTEM

🟪🟦🟧🟥

bactericidal > arteries, stimulates circulation, vasodilatory

SKIN, MUSCLES AND BODY TISSUES

🟦🟪🟦🟨🟥

antifungal, antiinflammatory, antiseptic, irritant, tissue toner > acne, athlete's foot, cellulite, eliminates lactic acid, fleas, pests, tired legs

RESPIRATORY SYSTEM

DIGESTIVE SYSTEM

🟦🟪🟦🟥

tonic > flatulence, liver

URINARY SYSTEM

🟦🟧🟥

diuretic >

REPRODUCTIVE SYSTEM

🟦

stimulates secretions > stimulates milk flow

CAUTIONS

Possible skin irritation.

BOTANICAL FAMILY

Gramineae: this family generally aids aches and pains and stimulates circulation.

Grass: distilled fresh partially dried leaves : sweet strong lemon aroma : top note. Used in traditional Indian medicine for fevers and infections also considered to be a sedative to the central nervous system. Might arrest growth of tumours.

Chemical constituents may include:

🟪 citral
🟦 methyl heptenone

🟧 limonene, dipentene
🟥 borneol, geraniol, nerol, farnesol, terpineol

# LEMONGRASS WEST INDIAN
## Cymbopogon citratus

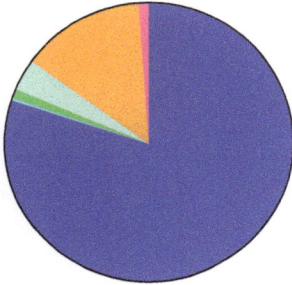

| | | |
|---|---|---|
| 🟦 | esters | yes |
| 🟪 | aliphatic aldehydes | 80.0% |
| ⬜ | ketones | 0.3% |
| 🟩 | sesquiterpenes | 1.0% |
| 🟩 | remainder | 3.7% |
| 🟨 | acids | yes |
| 🟧 | monoterpenes | 14.0% |
| 🟥 | alcohols | 1.0% |

## BODY SYSTEMS

NERVOUS SYSTEM

ENDOCRINE SYSTEM

CIRCULATION AND IMMUNE SYSTEM

SKIN, MUSCLES AND BODY TISSUES

RESPIRATORY SYSTEM

DIGESTIVE SYSTEM

URINARY SYSTEM

REPRODUCTIVE SYSTEM

CAUTIONS

BOTANICAL FAMILY

## PROPERTIES > USES

sedative, uplifting > depression

milk flow, reduces sweating, stimulates secretions > stimulates para-sympathetic nerves

bactericidal > arteries, stimulates circulation, vasodilatory

antifungal, antiinflammatory, antiseptic, calming, irritant, tissue toner > acne, athlete's foot, cellulite, eliminates lactic acid, fleas, pests, tired legs

tonic > flatulence, liver

diuretic >

stimulates secretions > stimulates milk flow

Possible skin irritation.

Gramineae: this family generally aids aches and pains and stimulates circulation.

Grass: distilled fresh partially dried leaves : sweet strong lemon aroma : top note. Used in traditional Indian medicine for fevers and infections also considered to be a sedative to the central nervous system. Might arrest growth of tumours.

Chemical constituents may include:

🟪 citral
⬜ methyl heptenone

🟧 mycrene, dipentene
🟥 linalool, geraniol, nerol, citronellol, farnesol

# LIME
## Citrus aurantifolia

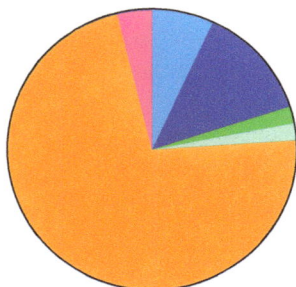

| | | |
|---|---|---|
| ■ | esters | 7.0% |
| ■ | aliphatic aldehydes | 13.0% |
| ■ | sesquiterpenes | yes |
| ■ | lactones and coumarins | 2.0% |
| ■ | remainder | 2.0% |
| ■ | oxides | yes |
| ■ | monoterpenes | 72.0% |
| ■ | alcohols | 4.0% |

## BODY SYSTEMS

**NERVOUS SYSTEM**
■ ■ ■ ■ ■ ■

**ENDOCRINE SYSTEM**
■ ■

**CIRCULATION AND IMMUNE SYSTEM**
■ ■ ■ ■ ■ ■

**SKIN, MUSCLES AND BODY TISSUES**
■ ■ ■ ■ ■ ■ ■

**RESPIRATORY SYSTEM**
■ ■ ■ ■ ■ ■

**DIGESTIVE SYSTEM**
■ ■ ■ ■ ■

**URINARY SYSTEM**

**REPRODUCTIVE SYSTEM**

CAUTIONS

BOTANICAL FAMILY

## PROPERTIES > USES

antispasmodic, sedative > anxiety, stress

temperature control > cooling

anticoagulant, antiviral, bactericidal, lowers blood pressure, tonic > stems bleeding
antiinflammatory, antiseptic, phototoxic > possible irritant, rheumatism, scurvy
decongestant, mucolytic > catarrh, sinusitis

stimulant > calms digestion, stimulates appetite

Phototoxic.

Rutaceae: this family generally aids digestion and skin.

Tree: cold expression of peel of unripe fruit : fresh sweet aroma : top note.
Lime oil that is distilled from the crushed fruit contains lower percentages of esters and aldehydes and only traces, if that, of the coumarins. Distilled oil has a sharp fresh aroma.

Chemical constituents may include:

■ geranyl acetate, methyl anthranilate
■ citral
■ bisabolene

■ bergaptene, limettin
■ limonene, pinenes, camphene, terpinolene, sabinene, p-cymene, myrcene
■ a-terpineol, linalool

# MANDARIN
## Citrus reticulata

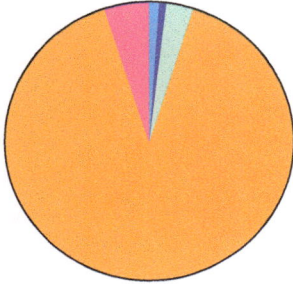

| | | |
|---|---|---|
| ⬜ | esters | 1.0% |
| 🟦 | aliphatic aldehydes | 1.0% |
| 🟩 | lactones and coumarins | yes |
| 🟩 | remainder | 3.0% |
| 🟧 | monoterpenes | 90.0% |
| 🟥 | alcohols | 5.0% |
| 🟧 | phenols, phe. ethers | yes |

## BODY SYSTEMS

NERVOUS SYSTEM

ENDOCRINE SYSTEM

CIRCULATION AND IMMUNE SYSTEM

SKIN, MUSCLES AND BODY TISSUES

RESPIRATORY SYSTEM

DIGESTIVE SYSTEM

URINARY SYSTEM

REPRODUCTIVE SYSTEM

NOTE

BOTANICAL FAMILY

## PROPERTIES > USES

antispasmodic, revitalising > anxiety, insomnia

stimulates secretions > balances metabolic rate, bile

antiviral, tonic >

antiseptic, cell regenerator > excellent for stretch marks

calming > breaks down fats, flatulence, improves bile production, liver

Especially good for children, women and elderly.

Rutaceae: this family generally aids digestion and skin.

Tree: cold expression of the outer peel : sweet sharp floral aroma : top note.
This fruit was given to the Mandarins as a mark of respect – hence its name.

Chemical constituents may include:

🟦 methyl anthranilate
🟦 decanal, sinensal, citral, citronellal
🟧 g-terpinene, limonene, pinenes, myrcene, p-cymene

🟥 linalool, citronellol, octanol
🟧 thymol

# MARJORAM SPANISH
## Thymus mastichina

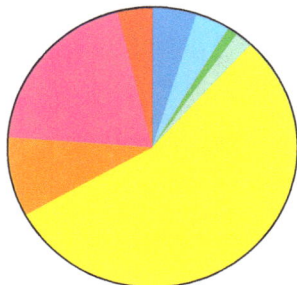

| | | |
|---|---|---|
| ■ | esters | 5.0% |
| ■ | ketones | 4.0% |
| ■ | sesquiterpenes | 1.0% |
| ■ | remainder | 2.0% |
| ■ | oxides | 55.0% |
| ■ | monoterpenes | 9.0% |
| ■ | alcohols | 20.0% |
| ■ | phenols, phe. ethers | 4.0% |

## BODY SYSTEMS

**NERVOUS SYSTEM**
■ ■ ■

**ENDOCRINE SYSTEM**
■ ■ ■

**CIRCULATION AND IMMUNE SYSTEM**
■ ■ ■ ■

**SKIN, MUSCLES AND BODY TISSUES**
■ ■ ■ ■ ■

**RESPIRATORY SYSTEM**
■ ■ ■ ■ ■ ■

**DIGESTIVE SYSTEM**

**URINARY SYSTEM**

**REPRODUCTIVE SYSTEM**

BOTANICAL FAMILY

## PROPERTIES > USES

calming >

stimulates mucous glands, stimulates secretions >

bactericidal >

antiseptic >

decongestant, expectorant > stimulates mucous glands

Lamiaceae.

Herb: distilled dried flowering herb : musty herby aroma : middle note.
There is considerable confusion between species of oregano and marjoram. Spanish marjoram has a different botanical classification to the french marjoram.

Chemical constituents may include:

■ linalyl acetate, terpinyl acetate, trans-pinocarvyl acetate
■ camphor
■ b-caryophyllene, gurjunene
■ 1.8-cineole, caryophyllene oxide

■ a-pinene, b-pinene, a-terpinene, g-terpinene, limonene, p-cymene, terpinolene
■ linalool, a-terpineol, cis-thujanol, trans-thujanol, trans-pinocarveol
■ thymol

# MARJORAM SWEET
## Origanum majorana

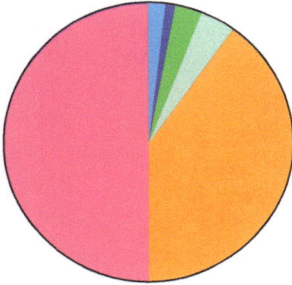

| | | |
|---|---|---|
| ■ | esters | 2.0% |
| ■ | aliphatic aldehydes | 1.0% |
| ■ | sesquiterpenes | 3.0% |
| ■ | remainder | 4.0% |
| ■ | monoterpenes | 44.0% |
| ■ | alcohols | 50.0% |
| ■ | phenols, phe. ethers | yes |

## BODY SYSTEMS

NERVOUS SYSTEM

ENDOCRINE SYSTEM

CIRCULATION AND IMMUNE SYSTEM

SKIN, MUSCLES AND BODY TISSUES

RESPIRATORY SYSTEM

DIGESTIVE SYSTEM

URINARY SYSTEM

REPRODUCTIVE SYSTEM

CAUTIONS

BOTANICAL FAMILY

## PROPERTIES > USES

analgesic, aphrodisiac, antispasmodic, balancing, calming > addiction, depression, headaches, obsessional, psychoses
balances > para-sympathetic nerves, under active thyroid
antiviral, bactericidal, lowers blood pressure > arteries, balances heart and circulation, vasodilatory
antifungal, antioxidant, antiseptic > arthritis, bruises (due to blood flow), cuts, muscle aches, rheumatism, toothache
bactericidal > bronchitis, catarrh, colds, coughs, nervous breathing, otitis, rhinitis, sinusitis
calming, diuretic > diarrhoea, enteritis, flatulence, laxative, ulcers

emmenagogue > painful periods, sexual obsession problems

Avoid during pregnancy.
Lamiaceae.

Herb: distilled flowering herb : spicy warm camphor like aroma : middle note.
Powerful effect for hyperactivity, calming to the nervous system excellent for deep emotional traumas – grief, loneliness etc. There are many species of marjoram with classification origanum – very difficult to identify and name. Known as 'joy of the mountain', given to married couples and planted in graveyards to bring peace to the departed.
Chemical constituents may include:

■ linalyl acetate, terpinyl acetate, geranyl acetate
■ citral
■ caryophyllene, cadinene

■ a-pinene, a-terpinene, g-terpinene, p-cymene, myrcene, limonene, ocimene, sabinene
■ linalool, borneol, a-terpineol, terpinen-4-ol
■ carvacrol, eugenol

51

# MELISSA LEMON BALM
## Melissa officinalis

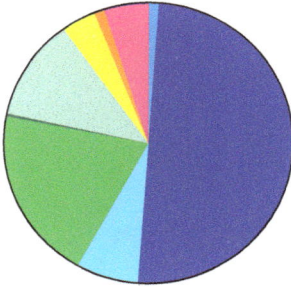

| | | |
|---|---|---|
| ☐ | esters | 1.2% |
| ☐ | aliphatic aldehydes | 50.0% |
| ☐ | ketones | 7.0% |
| ☐ | sesquiterpenes | 20.0% |
| ☐ | lactones and coumarins | yes |
| ☐ | remainder | 11.8% |
| ☐ | oxides | 4.0% |
| ☐ | monoterpenes | 1.0% |
| ☐ | alcohols | 5.0% |

## BODY SYSTEMS

**NERVOUS SYSTEM**
☐☐☐☐☐☐☐

**ENDOCRINE SYSTEM**
☐☐☐☐☐☐

**CIRCULATION AND IMMUNE SYSTEM**
☐☐☐☐☐

**SKIN, MUSCLES AND BODY TISSUES**
☐☐☐☐☐

**RESPIRATORY SYSTEM**
☐☐☐☐☐☐

**DIGESTIVE SYSTEM**
☐☐☐☐☐☐

**URINARY SYSTEM**

**REPRODUCTIVE SYSTEM**
☐☐☐

CAUTIONS

BOTANICAL FAMILY

## PROPERTIES > USES

antispasmodic, calming central system, hypnotic, sedative > depression, grief, headaches, hysteria, insomnia, vertigo

lowers fever, increases sweating > regulates heart, menstrual cycle and bile production

lowers blood pressure > anaemia, angina, irregular heart beat, palpitations

antiinflammatory, possible irritant > herpes (reduces healing time and lengthens time between attacks), wasp and bee stings

calming > allergies, rapid breathing

calming > cramps, indigestion, liver, nausea

uterine tonic >

Best avoided in pregnancy. Possible skin irritation. This oil is often adulterated.
Lamiaceae.

Herb: distilled leaves and flowering tops : sweet lemon flowery aroma : middle note. Famous for its calming effect on the heart and its rejuvenating effect. Found to be relaxant. Most melissa oils sold are blends of oils as true melissa is extremely expensive. Chemical constituents may include:

☐ geranyl acetate, neryl acetate, citronellyl acetate
☐ citronellal, citral
☐ methyl heptenone

☐ b-caryophyllene, germacrene, a-copaene
☐ 1.8-cineole, caryophyllene oxide
☐ limonene, trans-ocimene
☐ citronellol, geraniol, linalool

# MINT BERGAMOT
## Mentha citrata

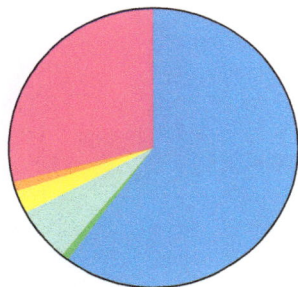

| | | |
|---|---|---|
| ■ | esters | 60.0% |
| ■ | aliphatic aldehydes | yes |
| ■ | sesquiterpenes | 0.9% |
| ■ | remainder | 6.2% |
| ■ | oxides | 3.0% |
| ■ | acids | yes |
| ■ | monoterpenes | 0.9% |
| ■ | alcohols | 29.0% |

## BODY SYSTEMS

**NERVOUS SYSTEM**

**ENDOCRINE SYSTEM**

**CIRCULATION AND IMMUNE SYSTEM**

**SKIN, MUSCLES AND BODY TISSUES**

**RESPIRATORY SYSTEM**

**DIGESTIVE SYSTEM**

**URINARY SYSTEM**

**REPRODUCTIVE SYSTEM**

## BOTANICAL FAMILY

## PROPERTIES > USES

antispasmodic, tonic > nervous exhaustion, soothing

balancing > stimulates liver and pancreas secretions

slightly bactericidal > heart regulation

slightly antiseptic, parasiticide > soothing

parasiticide, stimulates secretions > gastric, liver, pancreas

bactericidal > cystitis

tonic > impotence, stimulates ovaries

Lamiaceae.

Herb: distilled leaves and flowering tops : lemony mint aroma : middle note.
This mint has a high proportion of esters making it a gentler oil, excellent for balancing the body.

Chemical constituents may include:

■ linalyl acetate, geranyl acetate
■ caryophyllene, germacrene
■ 1.8-cineole, cis-linalool oxide, trans-linalool oxide
■ b-pinene
■ linalool, a-terpineol, citronellol, geraniol

# MINT CORNMINT
## Mentha arvensis

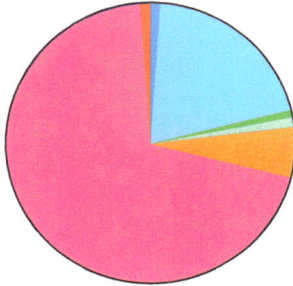

| | | |
|---|---|---|
| | esters | 1.0% |
| | aliphatic aldehydes | yes |
| | ketones | 20.0% |
| | sesquiterpenes | 1.0% |
| | lactones and coumarins | yes |
| | remainder | 1.0% |
| | oxides | yes |
| | acids | yes |
| | monoterpenes | 6.0% |
| | alcohols | 70.0% |
| | phenols, phe. ethers | 1.0% |

## BODY SYSTEMS

**NERVOUS SYSTEM**

**ENDOCRINE SYSTEM**

**CIRCULATION AND IMMUNE SYSTEM**

**SKIN, MUSCLES AND BODY TISSUES**

**RESPIRATORY SYSTEM**

**DIGESTIVE SYSTEM**

**URINARY SYSTEM**

**REPRODUCTIVE SYSTEM**

CAUTIONS

BOTANICAL FAMILY

## PROPERTIES > USES

anaesthetic, antispasmodic, stimulant, tonic > agitation, depression, migraine, motor nerves, sciatica, trembling

stimulates secretions > digestive juices, bile, gastric

bactericidal > energises heart

antiseptic, antimicrobic > eczema, possible irritation, toothache

expectorant > laryngitis, rhinitis, sinusitis

bactericidal > flatulence, indigestion, liver, ulcers, vomiting, worms

tonic > kidney, nephritis

Not for children under three years. Check for dermal irritation.

Lamiaceae.

Herb: distilled flowering herb : sweet bitter minty aroma : top note.
Many practitioners prefer peppermint oil because commercial cornmint oil is often fractionated. Chinese medicine uses cornmint for earache, tumours and skin conditions.
Chemical constituents may include:

- menthyl acetate
- menthone, isomenthone, piperitone, thujone
- caryophyllene
- menthofuran
- limonene, pinene, phellandrene
- menthol

# MINT PEPPERMINT
## Mentha piperita

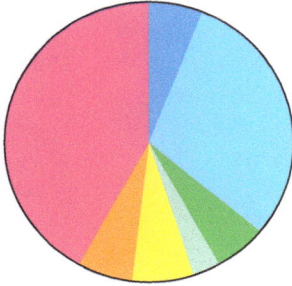

| | | |
|---|---|---|
| ☐ | esters | 6.0% |
| ☐ | aliphatic aldehydes | yes |
| ☐ | ketones | 30.0% |
| ☐ | sesquiterpenes | 6.0% |
| ☐ | lactones and coumarins | yes |
| ☐ | remainder | 3.0% |
| ☐ | oxides | 7.0% |
| ☐ | acids | yes |
| ☐ | monoterpenes | 6.0% |
| ☐ | alcohols | 42.0% |

## BODY SYSTEMS

NERVOUS SYSTEM
☐☐☐☐☐☐☐☐

ENDOCRINE SYSTEM
☐☐☐☐☐☐☐☐

CIRCULATION AND IMMUNE SYSTEM
☐☐☐☐

SKIN, MUSCLES AND BODY TISSUES
☐☐☐☐☐☐☐☐

RESPIRATORY SYSTEM
☐☐☐☐☐☐☐☐

DIGESTIVE SYSTEM
☐☐☐☐☐☐☐☐

URINARY SYSTEM
☐☐☐☐☐☐☐☐

REPRODUCTIVE SYSTEM
☐☐☐☐☐

CAUTIONS

BOTANICAL FAMILY

## PROPERTIES > USES

anaesthetic, analgesic, antispasmodic, tonic > mental fatigue, migraine, nervous trembling, sciatica
balancing, lowers fever, reduces milk production, lowers temperature > nervous system and menstrual cycle, stimulates heart and ovaries
antiviral, bactericidal, raises blood pressure > constricts capillaries
antifungal, antiinflammatory, antiseptic > asthma, eczema, gnats, herpes, rashes, ringworm, yellow fever
expectorant, mucolytic > bronchitis, laryngitis, otitis, rhinitis, sinusitis
tonic > cirrhosis, enteritis, gall stones, hepatitis, jaundice, liver, travel sickness, ulcers, vomiting, worms
bactericidal > cystitis, nephritis, prostate

uterine tonic > assists childbirth, impotence, reduces milk production

Not for use in pregnancy or with nursing mothers or with children under three years old.
Lamiaceae.

Herb: distilled leaves and flowering tops : piercing menthol aroma : top note.
Excellent for digestive problems and for local anaesthetic for wounds. Romans were well aware of its detoxifying properties and wore crowns of the herb at feasts. Used for irritable bowel syndrome.
Chemical constituents may include:

☐ menthyl acetate
☐ menthone, isomenthone, pulegone
☐ germacrene, b-caryophyllene
☐ aesculetine, menthofuran

☐ 1.8-cineole, caryophyllene oxide
☐ phellandrene, a-pinene, b-pinene, menthene, limonene
☐ menthol, neomenthol, isomenthol, linalool

55

# MINT SPEARMINT
## Mentha spicata

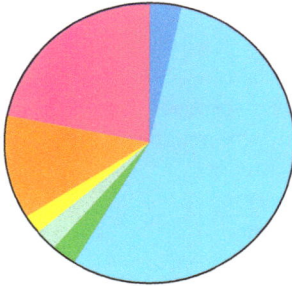

| | | |
|---|---|---|
| ■ | esters | 3.5% |
| ■ | ketones | 55.0% |
| ■ | sesquiterpenes | 3.0% |
| ■ | remainder | 2.3% |
| ■ | oxides | 2.2% |
| ■ | acids | yes |
| ■ | monoterpenes | 12.0% |
| ■ | alcohols | 22.0% |

## BODY SYSTEMS

NERVOUS SYSTEM
■ ■ ■ ■ ■ ■

ENDOCRINE SYSTEM
■ ■ ■

CIRCULATION AND IMMUNE SYSTEM
■ ■ ■ ■ ■

SKIN, MUSCLES AND BODY TISSUES
■ ■ ■ ■ ■ ■

RESPIRATORY SYSTEM
■ ■ ■ ■ ■

DIGESTIVE SYSTEM
■ ■ ■ ■ ■ ■

URINARY SYSTEM
■ ■ ■ ■ ■ ■

REPRODUCTIVE SYSTEM

## PROPERTIES > USES

calming, local anaesthetic, tonic > headaches, fatigue, migraine, nervous exhaustion, stress

lowers fever, stimulates bile secretions >

decongestant, astringent >

antiseptic, strongly antiinflammatory > congested skin, wounds

expectorant, mucolytic > bronchitis, fevers, flu, sinusitis

tonic > bile flow, dyspepsia, flatulence, liver, vomiting

diuretic > cystitis

CAUTIONS — Avoid in pregnancy and with young children.

BOTANICAL FAMILY — Lamiaceae.

Herb: distilled flowering tops : spicy warm minty aroma : top note.
Valued highly as a culinary herb. The water from distillation is used to relieve coughs, colic, hiccoughs and flatulence.

Chemical constituents may include:

■ cis-carvyl acetate, trans-carvyl acetate, dihydrocarvyl acetate
■ carvone, dihydrocarvone, menthone
■ caryophyllene, elemene, farnesene, bourbonene

■ 1,8-cineole
■ limonene, a-pinene, b-pinene phellandrene, camphene
■ linalool, menthol

# MYRRH
## Commiphora molmol

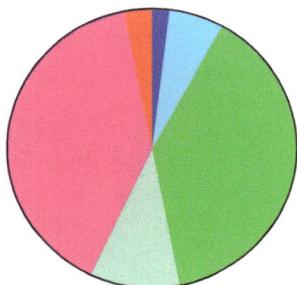

| | | |
|---|---|---|
| 🟦 | esters | yes |
| 🟪 | aliphatic aldehydes | 2.0% |
| 🟦 | ketones | 6.0% |
| 🟩 | sesquiterpenes | 39.0% |
| 🟩 | remainder | 10.0% |
| 🟨 | acids | yes |
| 🟫 | aromatic aldehydes | yes |
| 🟧 | monoterpenes | yes |
| 🟥 | alcohols | 40.0% |
| 🟧 | phenols, phe. ethers | 3.0% |

## BODY SYSTEMS

NERVOUS SYSTEM

ENDOCRINE SYSTEM

CIRCULATION AND IMMUNE SYSTEM

SKIN, MUSCLES AND BODY TISSUES

RESPIRATORY SYSTEM

DIGESTIVE SYSTEM

URINARY SYSTEM

REPRODUCTIVE SYSTEM

## PROPERTIES > USES

calming > deodorant, sexual stimulus, weakness

hormone like, temperature control > glandular fever, overactive thyroid

antiviral, astringent, bactericidal, immune system tonic > stimulates white corpuscles

antifungal, antiinflammatory, antiseptic > athlete's foot, bedsores, gangrene, herpes, ringworm, ulcers, wet eczema

antiseptic > bronchitis, drying nature excellent for pulmonary infections

tonic > diarrhoea, haemorrhoids, hepatitis

diuretic >

emmenagogue > amenorrhoea, leucorrhoea, thrush

CAUTIONS — Best avoided in pregnancy.
BOTANICAL FAMILY — Buseraceae.
Tree: solvent extraction of crude myrrh to give a resinoid or steam distillation of the crude myrrh to give an essential oil : musky smoky aroma : base note.
Excellent for all septic skin conditions. Used in embalming.
Chemical constituents may include:

- 🟦 myrrholic ester
- 🟪 2-butanal
- 🟦 methyl isobutyl ketone, curzerenone
- 🟩 elemene, heerabolene, cadinene, copaene, curzerene, lindestrene
- 🟨 myrrholic acid
- 🟫 cinnamaldehyde, cuminaldehyde
- 🟨 limonene, dipentene, pinene
- 🟥 myrrh alcohols
- 🟧 eugenol

# NIAOULI
## Melaleuca viridiflora

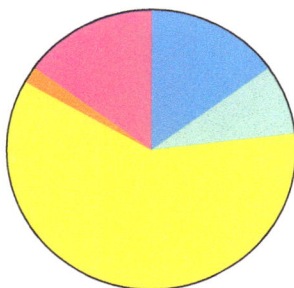

| | | |
|---|---|---|
| 🟦 | esters | 15.0% |
| 🟪 | aliphatic aldehydes | yes |
| 🟩 | sesquiterpenes | yes |
| ⬜ | remainder | 8.0% |
| 🟨 | oxides | 60.0% |
| 🟫 | aromatic aldehydes | yes |
| 🟧 | monoterpenes | 2.0% |
| 🟥 | alcohols | 15.0% |

## BODY SYSTEMS

NERVOUS SYSTEM

ENDOCRINE SYSTEM

CIRCULATION AND IMMUNE SYSTEM

SKIN, MUSCLES AND BODY TISSUES

RESPIRATORY SYSTEM

DIGESTIVE SYSTEM

URINARY SYSTEM

REPRODUCTIVE SYSTEM

BOTANICAL FAMILY

## PROPERTIES > USES

analgesic, stimulant > aids concentration, clarifying

lowers fever, oestrogen like >

strongly antiviral, bactericidal, decongestant, immune system tonic > increases antibodies, HIV
antiseptic, tissue toner > acne, aches and pains, boils, burns, radiography burns, rheumatism, spots, ulcers
bactericidal > asthma, bronchitis, catarrh, coughs, pneumonia, sinusitis, sore throat
tonic > enteritis, gastric and duodenal ulcers, intestinal parasites
bactericidal > cystitis

antiviral > fibroids, genital herpes, leucorrhea, prostate

Myrtaceae: this family is generally stimulating and good for the respiratory system.

Tree: distilled leaves and shoots : sweet clear penetrating aroma : top note.
Falling leaves cause healthy atmosphere due to strong disinfectant properties.
Recommended for serious conditions such as aids and nonhormonal cancer.

Chemical constituents may include:
- 🟦 terpinyl valerate, terpinyl acetate, terpinyl butyrate isovaleraldehyde
- 🟪 isovaleraldehyde
- 🟩 b-carophyllene, viridiflorene
- 🟨 1.8-cineole
- 🟫 benzaldehyde
- 🟧 limonene, a-pinene, b-pinene
- 🟥 a-terpineol, viridiflorol, nerolidol, globulol

# NUTMEG
## Myristica fragrans

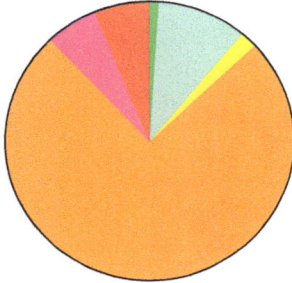

| | | |
|---|---|---|
| 🟩 | sesquiterpenes | 1.0% |
| 🟦 | remainder | 10.0% |
| 🟨 | oxides | 2.0% |
| 🟧 | acids | yes |
| 🟧 | monoterpenes | 75.0% |
| 🟥 | alcohols | 6.0% |
| 🟧 | phenols, phe. ethers | 6.0% |

## BODY SYSTEMS

**NERVOUS SYSTEM**

**ENDOCRINE SYSTEM**

**CIRCULATION AND IMMUNE SYSTEM**

**SKIN, MUSCLES AND BODY TISSUES**

**RESPIRATORY SYSTEM**

**DIGESTIVE SYSTEM**

**URINARY SYSTEM**

**REPRODUCTIVE SYSTEM**

CAUTIONS

BOTANICAL FAMILY

## PROPERTIES > USES

antispasmodic, tonic > excites motor cortex, neuralgia, Raynaud's disease

oestrogen like >

bactericidal > invigorating to heart and circulation

antiseptic, parasiticide > good for hair, haemorrhoids, rhuematism, sprains, toothache

stimulant > diarrhoea, digestion of heavy foods, gall stones

emmenagogue, uterine tonic > assists childbirth, frigidity, impotence, scanty periods

Treat with care the myristicin can cause hallucinations. Avoid in pregnancy.

Myristicaceae.

Tree: distilled fruits : sharp, aroma : top note.
A nutmeg is like a small peach, the oil comes from the kernel. Oil obtained from the husk is called mace and contains even more myristicin. Nutmeg was traditionally used for stomach disorders. Nutmeg inhibits platelet aggregation.

Chemical constituents may include:
🟩 b-caryophyllene
🟨 1.8-cineole
🟧 a-pinene, b-pinene, a-terpinene, g-terpinene, sabinene, myrcene, limonene, camphene, dipentene, p-cymene

🟥 terpinen-4-ol, a-terpineol, linalool, borneol, geraniol
🟧 myristicin, elemicin, safrole, eugenol

# ORANGE BITTER
## Citrus aurantium amara

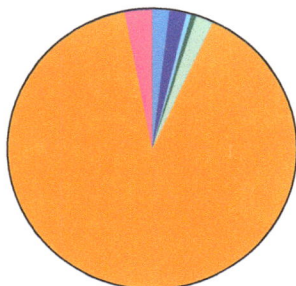

| | | |
|---|---|---|
| 🟦 | esters | 2.0% |
| 🟦 | aliphatic aldehydes | 2.0% |
| 🟦 | ketones | yes |
| 🟩 | sesquiterpenes | 0.5% |
| 🟩 | lactones and coumarins | 0.5% |
| 🟦 | remainder | 2.0% |
| 🟨 | oxides | yes |
| 🟧 | acids | yes |
| 🟧 | monoterpenes | 90.0% |
| 🟥 | alcohols | 3.0% |

## BODY SYSTEMS

NERVOUS SYSTEM

🟦🟦🟦🟩🟩🟨🟧🟥

ENDOCRINE SYSTEM

CIRCULATION AND IMMUNE SYSTEM

🟦🟩🟩🟨🟧🟥

SKIN, MUSCLES AND BODY TISSUES

🟦🟦🟦🟩🟩🟨🟧🟥

RESPIRATORY SYSTEM

DIGESTIVE SYSTEM

🟦🟦🟦🟩🟩🟧🟥

URINARY SYSTEM

REPRODUCTIVE SYSTEM

CAUTIONS

BOTANICAL FAMILY

## PROPERTIES > USES

calming, cheering, stimulating > anxiety, vertigo

anticoagulant, bactericidal, astringent > circulation

antiaging, antifungal, antiinflammatory, antiseptic, cell regenerator, phototoxic, tonic >

calming > nervous indigestion, liver stimulant, constipation

Use with care skin may photosensitive after application.

Rutaceae: this family generally aids digestion and skin problems.

Tree: cold expression almost ripe peel : strong pervasive orange aroma : top note. Both oranges and lemons have been used traditionally to treat palpitations, to thin the blood and to cure scurvy.

Chemical constituents may include:

🟦 linalyl acetate, geranyl acetate, citronellyl acetate

🟦 undecanal, citral

🟩 farnesene, copaene, humulene

🟩 auraptene, bergaptene, limettin

🟨 1.8-cineole

🟧 limonene, a-pinene, myrcene, terpinolene, camphene, p-cymene, ocimene

🟥 linalool, nerol, a-terpineol, citronellol

# ORANGE BLOSSOM NEROLI
## Citrus aurantium amara

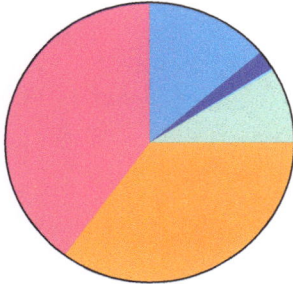

| | | |
|---|---|---|
| ■ | esters | 14.0% |
| ■ | aliphatic aldehydes | 2.0% |
| ■ | ketones | 0.5% |
| ■ | sesquiterpenes | yes |
| ■ | remainder | 8.5% |
| ■ | acids | yes |
| ■ | monoterpenes | 35.0% |
| ■ | alcohols | 40.0% |

## BODY SYSTEMS

NERVOUS SYSTEM

ENDOCRINE SYSTEM

CIRCULATION AND IMMUNE SYSTEM

SKIN, MUSCLES AND BODY TISSUES

RESPIRATORY SYSTEM

DIGESTIVE SYSTEM

URINARY SYSTEM

REPRODUCTIVE SYSTEM

BOTANICAL FAMILY

## PROPERTIES > USES

analgesic, aphrodisiac, antispasmodic > peace inducing, revitalising
balancing > menopause, pmt

bactericidal, lowers blood pressure, tonic > phlebitis, ulcers, varicose veins
antiaging, antifungal, cell generator > deodorant, protection from radiography burns, rheumatism
bactericidal > bronchitis, TB

calming, tonic > diabetes, haemorrhoids, liver, pancreas

uterine tonic > menopause, pmt

Rutaceae: this family generally aids digestion and skin problems.

Tree: distilled freshly picked flowers : haunting and beautiful aroma : base note.
Very powerful for emotional problems. Used by Italian Countess of Neroli, Anne Marie, to perfume her gloves and bathing water – hence the name. Good antifungal activities.

Chemical constituents may include:

■ methyl anthranilate, linalyl acetate, geranyl acetate, neryl acetate
■ jasmone
■ indole
■ phenylacetic acid
■ limonene, b-pinene
■ linalool, a-terpineol, geraniol, nerol, nerolidol, farnesol, benzyl alcohol, phenylether alcohol

# ORANGE PETITGRAIN
## Citrus aurantium amara

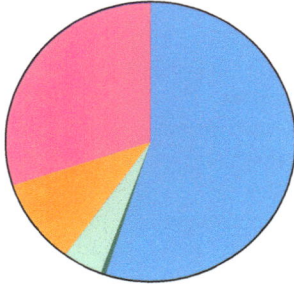

| | | |
|---|---|---|
| ■ | esters | 55.0% |
| ■ | aliphatic aldehydes | yes |
| ■ | lactones and coumarins | 0.5% |
| ■ | remainder | 4.5% |
| ■ | acids | yes |
| ■ | monoterpenes | 10.0% |
| ■ | alcohols | 30.0% |
| ■ | phenols, phe. ethers | yes |

## BODY SYSTEMS

NERVOUS SYSTEM
■ ■ ■ ■ ■ ■
ENDOCRINE SYSTEM

CIRCULATION AND IMMUNE SYSTEM
■ ■ ■

SKIN, MUSCLES AND BODY TISSUES
■ ■ ■ ■ ■ ■ ■
RESPIRATORY SYSTEM
■ ■ ■ ■ ■ ■ ■
DIGESTIVE SYSTEM
■ ■ ■ ■ ■ ■
URINARY SYSTEM

REPRODUCTIVE SYSTEM

BOTANICAL FAMILY

## PROPERTIES > USES

antispasmodic, calming, cheering > depression, nervous exhaustion

bactericidal > slight stimulation of immune system

antifungal, antioxidant, antiseptic, deodorant > infected acne, rheumatism (nervous)
tonic > bronchitis

calming > flatulence, nervous indigestion

Rutaceae: this family generally aids digestion and skin problems.

Tree: distilled leaves and twigs : woody floral aroma : top note.
Classic ingredient of eau-de-cologne and widely used as a food flavouring. Good antifungal agent.

Chemical constituents may include:

■ linalyl acetate, geranyl acetate, neryl acetate
■ citral
■ limettin, bergaptene

■ a-pinene, limonene, p-cymene, ocimene, myrcene
■ linalool, geraniol, nerolidol, a-terpineol
■ thymol

# ORANGE SWEET
## Citrus sinensis

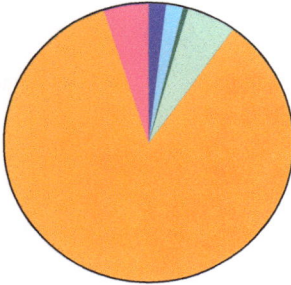

| | | |
|---|---|---|
| aliphatic aldehydes | 2.0% |
| ketones | 2.0% |
| sesquiterpenes | yes |
| lactones and coumarins | 0.5% |
| remainder | 5.5% |
| acids | yes |
| monoterpenes | 85.0% |
| alcohols | 5.0% |

**BODY SYSTEMS**

**PROPERTIES > USES**

NERVOUS SYSTEM

sedative, warming > depression, nervous tension

ENDOCRINE SYSTEM

stimulates secretions > bile

CIRCULATION AND IMMUNE SYSTEM

bactericidal, lowers blood pressure, stimulant > colds, flu, fluid retention, obesity

SKIN, MUSCLES AND BODY TISSUES

antifungal (22), antiinflammatory, antiseptic > dull complexion, mouth ulcers

RESPIRATORY SYSTEM

bactericidal, decongestant > bronchitis, chills

DIGESTIVE SYSTEM

carminative, tonic > bile flow, constipation, indigestion

URINARY SYSTEM

REPRODUCTIVE SYSTEM

BOTANICAL FAMILY

Rutaceae: this family generally aids digestion and skin problems.

Tree: cold expression of fresh peel or distilled fresh peel : lingering rich fruity aroma if expressed, a lighter aroma if distilled : top note.
Dried sweet orange peel is used in Chinese medicine.

Chemical constituents may include:

decanal, citronellal, octanal

carvone, a-ionone

bergaptene, auraptene

limonene, myrcene, sabinene, a-pinene

linalool, a-terpineol, geraniol

# ORIGANUM
## Origanum heracleoticum carvacroliferum

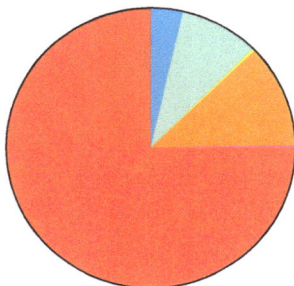

| | | |
|---|---|---|
| 🟦 | esters | 3.5% |
| 🟩 | sesquiterpenes | yes |
| ⬜ | remainder | 9.0% |
| 🟨 | oxides | 0.3% |
| 🟧 | acids | yes |
| 🟧 | monoterpenes | 12.0% |
| 🟪 | alcohols | 0.2% |
| 🟥 | phenols, phe. ethers | 75.0% |

## BODY SYSTEMS

NERVOUS SYSTEM

ENDOCRINE SYSTEM

CIRCULATION AND IMMUNE SYSTEM

SKIN, MUSCLES AND BODY TISSUES

RESPIRATORY SYSTEM

DIGESTIVE SYSTEM

URINARY SYSTEM

REPRODUCTIVE SYSTEM

CAUTIONS

BOTANICAL FAMILY

## PROPERTIES > USES

analgesic, antispasmodic, stimulant, tonic > neuralgia

increases sweating > warming

antiviral, bactericidal > increases leucocyte activity, tonic to immune system

antifungal, antiseptic, parasiticide > rheumatism, skin irritation possible

expectorant > bronchitis, irritation of mucous membrane possible

carminative > aerophagy (swallowing gulps of air), flatulence, worms

diuretic >

emmenagogue >

Avoid in pregnancy. Use with extreme care due to high percentage of phenols.

Lamiaceae.

Herb: distilled dried flowering tops : herbaceous tarry refreshing aroma : middle note. Properties similar to common thyme (thymus vulgaris) and wild origanum (origanum vulgare) but has much higher percentage of phenols.

Chemical constituents may include:

🟦 linalyl acetate
🟩 caryophyllene
🟨 1.8-cineole

🟧 a-terpinene, g-terpinene, p-cymene
🟪 linalool
🟥 carvacrol, thymol

# PALMAROSA
## Cymbopogon martinii

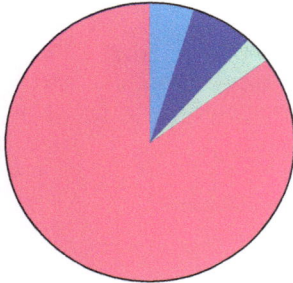

| | | |
|---|---|---|
| ■ | esters | 5.0% |
| ■ | aliphatic aldehydes | 7.0% |
| □ | ketones | yes |
| ■ | sesquiterpenes | yes |
| ■ | remainder | 3.0% |
| ■ | monoterpenes | yes |
| ■ | alcohols | 85.0% |

## BODY SYSTEMS

**NERVOUS SYSTEM**
■ ■ □ ■ ■ ■

**ENDOCRINE SYSTEM**
■ □ ■ ■

**CIRCULATION AND IMMUNE SYSTEM**
■ □ ■ ■ ■

**SKIN, MUSCLES AND BODY TISSUES**
■ ■ □ ■ ■ ■

**RESPIRATORY SYSTEM**
■ ■ □ ■ ■ ■

**DIGESTIVE SYSTEM**
■ ■ □ ■ ■

**URINARY SYSTEM**
■ ■ □ ■ ■

**REPRODUCTIVE SYSTEM**
■ ■

## BOTANICAL FAMILY

## PROPERTIES > USES

calming, cheering, tonic > nervous exhaustion

lowers fever, stimulates sebum production >
balances fluid retention

strongly antiviral, antimicrobic, strongly
bactericidal, tonic > cardiac

strongly antifungal, antiseptic, cell generator > acne,
dry cracked skin, dry and wet eczema, eases stiff joints

bactericidal > bronchitis, rhinitis, sinusitis

stimulant > anorexia, enteritis

bactericidal > cystitis

uterine tonic > assists childbirth, cervix, uterus,
vagina

Gramineae: this family generally aids aches and
pains and stimulates circulation.

Grass: distilled leaves : sweet dry rose like aroma : top note.
Known as Indian geranium oil, ginger grass is a chemotype of palmarosa. Often used to
adulterate rose oil.

Chemical constituents may include:
- ■ geranyl acetate, geranyl formate, geranyl isobutyrate, geranyl hexanoate, neryl formate
- ■ citral, citronellal
- □ methyl heptenone
- ■ b-caryophyllene
- ■ dipentene, limonene
- ■ geraniol, citronellol, farnesol, linalool, nerol, elemol

# PATCHOULI
## Pogostemon cablin

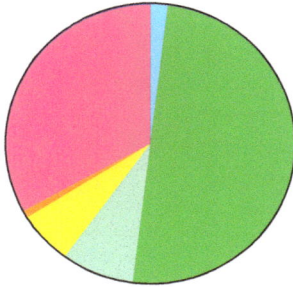

| | | |
|---|---|---|
| ketones | 2.0% |
| sesquiterpenes | 50.0% |
| remainder | 8.0% |
| oxides | 6.0% |
| acids | yes |
| monoterpenes | 1.0% |
| alcohols | 30.0% |

## BODY SYSTEMS

NERVOUS SYSTEM

ENDOCRINE SYSTEM

CIRCULATION AND IMMUNE SYSTEM

SKIN, MUSCLES AND BODY TISSUES

RESPIRATORY SYSTEM

DIGESTIVE SYSTEM

URINARY SYSTEM

REPRODUCTIVE SYSTEM

BOTANICAL FAMILY

## PROPERTIES > USES

aphrodisiac, balancing, calming, tonic > depression, makes mind more objective
lowers fever >

antiviral, astringent, bactericidal, decongestant, tonic to immune system > phlebitis, varicose veins
antifungal, antiinflammatory, antiseptic, cell generator > acne, athlete's foot, eczema, insects, loose or dry skin

carminative > curbs appetite, diarrhoea, enteritis, haemorrhoids
diuretic >

Lamiaceae.

Herb: distilled fermented dried leaves : sweet earthy aroma : base note.
Oil matures with age. Excellent for dry cracked skin conditions.

Chemical constituents may include:

patchoulenone, isopatchoulenone
guaiene, patchoulenes, a-bulnesene, caryophyllene, aromadendrene

guaiene oxide, bulnesene oxide caryophyllene oxide
pinenes, limonene
guaiol, bulnesol, pogostol, patchouli alcohol

# PENNYROYAL
## Mentha pulegium

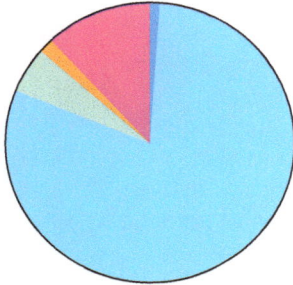

| | | |
|---|---|---|
| ■ | esters | 1.0% |
| ■ | ketones | 80.0% |
| ■ | remainder | 5.5% |
| ■ | monoterpenes | 1.5% |
| ■ | alcohols | 12.0% |

BODY SYSTEMS

PROPERTIES > USES

NERVOUS SYSTEM
■ ■

antispasmodic, neurotoxic >

ENDOCRINE SYSTEM
■ ■

lowers fever, causes sweating >

CIRCULATION AND IMMUNE SYSTEM
■ ■ ■

raises blood pressure > heart stimulant

SKIN, MUSCLES AND BODY TISSUES
■ ■ ■ ■

antiseptic > insect repellent

RESPIRATORY SYSTEM
■ ■ ■ ■

mucolytic > bronchitis, catarrh

DIGESTIVE SYSTEM
■ ■ ■ ■

carminative > flatulence, liver, spleen

URINARY SYSTEM

REPRODUCTIVE SYSTEM
■

abortive, emmenagogue > leucorrhoea

CAUTIONS

Avoid in pregnancy and young children. Use with great caution as ketones can accumulate in the body.

BOTANICAL FAMILY

Lamiaceae.

Herb: distilled fresh or slightly dried herb : minty herby aroma.
Still in the British Herbal Pharmacopoeia for flatulence, intestinal colic, cutaneous eruptions, gout and delayed periods. Not recommended by some practitioner.

Chemical constituents may include:

■ neoisomenthyl acetate
■ pulegone, menthone, piperite-none, trans-isopulegone

■ a-pinene. b-pinene, limonene
■ linalool, menthol, neomenthol, neoisomenthol

# PINE DWARF
## Pinus mugo turra

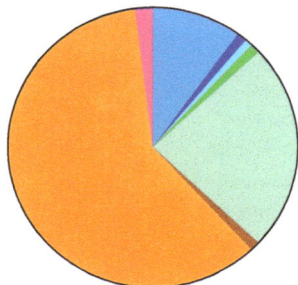

| | | |
|---|---|---|
| ■ | esters | 10.0% |
| ■ | aliphatic aldehydes | 1.0% |
| ■ | ketones | 1.0% |
| ■ | sesquiterpenes | 1.0% |
| ■ | remainder | 24.0% |
| ■ | aromatic aldehydes | 1.0% |
| ■ | monoterpenes | 60.0% |
| ■ | alcohols | 2.0% |

BODY SYSTEMS

NERVOUS SYSTEM
■ ■ ■ ■ ■ ■

ENDOCRINE SYSTEM
■

CIRCULATION AND IMMUNE SYSTEM
■ ■ ■ ■ ■ ■

SKIN, MUSCLES AND BODY TISSUES
■ ■ ■ ■ ■ ■

RESPIRATORY SYSTEM
■ ■ ■ ■ ■

DIGESTIVE SYSTEM

URINARY SYSTEM
■ ■ ■

REPRODUCTIVE SYSTEM

CAUTIONS

BOTANICAL FAMILY

PROPERTIES > USES

calming, cheering >

slightly hormone like > warming

slightly bactericidal, slightly antiviral, decongestant > arteries, circulation

slightly antiinflammatory, air antiseptic, irritant >

antiseptic, expectorant > bronchitis, pleurisy, sinusitis, TB

diuretic >

Use with care as skin irritation is likely. Some practitioners do not recommend the use of this oil. Pinaceae: this family is generally highly antiseptic and aids respiratory problems.

Tree: distilled needles and twigs : sweet soothing spicy woody unusual aroma due to aldehydes : middle note. The needles are used to make medical preparations for bladder, kidney and muscular pains also inhalents for respiratory problems.

Chemical constituents may include:
■ bornyl acetate, bornyl propionate, bornyl caproate
■ caproaldehyde
■ cryptone
■ cadinene

■ anisaldehyde, cuminaldehyde
■ carene, limonene, pinenes phellandrene, mrycene, camphene
■ pumiliol

# PINE LONGLEAF TURPENTINE

## Pinus palustris

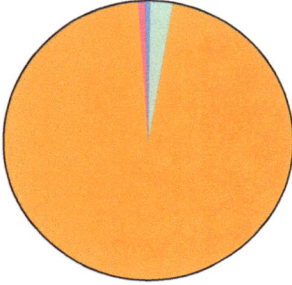

| | esters | 0.2% |
| --- | --- | --- |
| | remainder | 2.6% |
| | monoterpenes | 96.0% |
| | alcohols | 1.0% |
| | phenols, phe. ethers | 0.2% |

**BODY SYSTEMS**

**PROPERTIES > USES**

**NERVOUS SYSTEM**

analgesic, antispasmodic, stimulant, warming > sciatica

**ENDOCRINE SYSTEM**

**CIRCULATION AND IMMUNE SYSTEM**

bactericidal, tonic > arrests bleeding

**SKIN, MUSCLES AND BODY TISSUES**

antiseptic, parasiticide > arthritis, boils, cuts, fleas, muscular aches and pains, rheumatism, ringworm, scabies, wounds

**RESPIRATORY SYSTEM**

expectorant > bronchitis, catarrh, whooping cough

**DIGESTIVE SYSTEM**

**URINARY SYSTEM**

diuretic > cystitis, urethritis

**REPRODUCTIVE SYSTEM**

mucolytic > leucorrhoea

BOTANICAL FAMILY

Pinaceae: this family is generally highly antiseptic and aids respiratory problems.

Tree: distilled oleoresin from wood chips : warm soothing aroma : middle note. Used by Galen and Hippocrates. Used in China both internally and externally for hundreds of years. Most commonly used now for paint and stain remover but still used extensively in many ointments and lotions for aches and pains.

Chemical constituents may include:

- bornyl acetate
- pinenes
- borneol, pinocarveol, terpineol, fenchol
- methyl chavicol (estragole)

# PINE LONGLEAF WOOD
## Pinus palustris

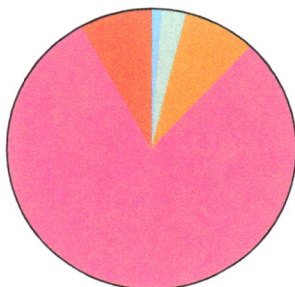

| | | |
|---|---|---|
| ☐ | ketones | 1.0% |
| ☐ | remainder | 2.9% |
| ☐ | oxides | 0.1% |
| ☐ | monoterpenes | 8.0% |
| ☐ | alcohols | 80.0% |
| ☐ | phenols, phe. ethers | 8.0% |

BODY SYSTEMS

PROPERTIES > USES

NERVOUS SYSTEM

analgesic, stimulant >

ENDOCRINE SYSTEM

CIRCULATION AND IMMUNE SYSTEM

bactericidal, decongestant > stimulates circulation

SKIN, MUSCLES AND BODY TISSUES

antiseptic, insecticide > arthritis, lumbago, rheumatism

RESPIRATORY SYSTEM

expectorant > asthma, bronchitis, catarrh, sinusitis

DIGESTIVE SYSTEM

URINARY SYSTEM

REPRODUCTIVE SYSTEM

BOTANICAL FAMILY

Pinaceae: this family is generally highly antiseptic and aids respiratory problems.

Tree: distilled heartwood : sweet soothing pine aroma : middle note.
Pine sawdust poultices have been used very successfully for rheumatism, hard cancerous deposits and lumbago.

Chemical constituents may include:

☐ fenchone
☐ pinenes

☐ terpineol, fenchol, borneol
☐ methyl chavicol (estragole)

# PINE SCOTCH
## Pinus sylvestris

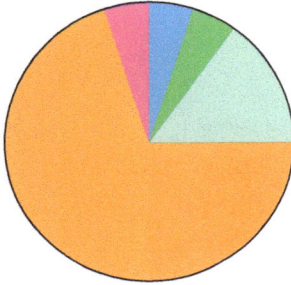

| | | |
|---|---|---|
| | esters | 5.0% |
| | aliphatic aldehydes | yes |
| | ketones | yes |
| | sesquiterpenes | 5.0% |
| | remainder | 15.0% |
| | oxides | yes |
| | acids | yes |
| | aromatic aldehydes | yes |
| | monoterpenes | 70.0% |
| | alcohols | 5.0% |
| | phenols, phe. ethers | yes |

## BODY SYSTEMS

NERVOUS SYSTEM

ENDOCRINE SYSTEM

CIRCULATION AND IMMUNE SYSTEM

SKIN, MUSCLES AND BODY TISSUES

RESPIRATORY SYSTEM

DIGESTIVE SYSTEM

URINARY SYSTEM

REPRODUCTIVE SYSTEM

CAUTIONS

BOTANICAL FAMILY

## PROPERTIES > USES

analgesic, aphrodisiac, stimulant, tonic > frigidity, impotence, multiple sclerosis

cortisone like, hormone like, temperature balancing > adrenal glands

bactericidal, decongestant, raises blood pressure > lymph system

antifungal, antiinflammatory, antiseptic > allergies, arthritis, eczema, muscular aches and pains, psoriasis

expectorant > asthma, excellent for bronchitis, sinusitis

stimulates secretions > diabetes, gall stones, gastric, hepatitis, indigestion

diuretic > cystitis

decongestant > fallopian tubes, ovaries, stimulates egg and sperm production, uterus

Use with care check sensitive skin for irritation.
Pinaceae: this family is generally highly antiseptic and aids respiratory problems.

Tree: distilled dry needles : fresh forest aroma : middle note.
It is acknowledged that the pine forests produce a healing environment due to the evaporation of the essential oil from the pine needles.
Chemical constituents may include:

- bornyl acetate, terpinyl acetate
- citronellal, citral
- cryptone
- caryophyllene, cadinene, copaene, guaiene, farnesene

- cuminaldehyde, anisaldehyde
- a-pinene, b-pinene, limonene, carene, camphene, phellandrene, dipentene, terpinenes, myrcene, sabinene
- borneol, terpinen-4-ol, cadinol

71

# RAVENSARA AROMATIC

## Ravensara aromatica

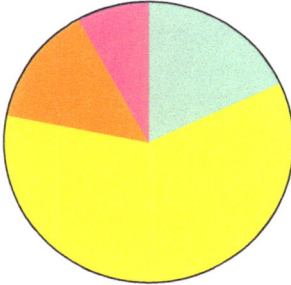

| | | |
|---|---|---|
| 🟦 | esters | yes |
| 🟩 | sesquiterpenes | yes |
| 🟢 | remainder | 18.0% |
| 🟨 | oxides | 60.0% |
| 🟧 | monoterpenes | 14.0% |
| 🟪 | alcohols | 8.0% |

## BODY SYSTEMS

NERVOUS SYSTEM
🟦🟩🟨🟧🟪

ENDOCRINE SYSTEM
🟨🟧🟪

CIRCULATION AND IMMUNE SYSTEM
🟩🟧🟪

SKIN, MUSCLES AND BODY TISSUES
🟦🟩🟧🟪

RESPIRATORY SYSTEM
🟦🟩🟨🟧🟪

DIGESTIVE SYSTEM
🟦🟩🟨🟧🟪

URINARY SYSTEM

REPRODUCTIVE SYSTEM

BOTANICAL FAMILY

## PROPERTIES > USES

tonic > dendritis, insomnia

tonic > glandular fever

antiviral, bactericidal >

antifungal, antiseptic > chicken pox, herpes, muscle aches and pains
expectorant > bronchitis, flu, sinusitis, whooping cough
stimulates secretions > enteritis, gastric, liver

Lauraceae: this family is usually powerful and stimulating.

Shrub: distilled foliage : clear aroma : middle note.
Relaxing to system when massaged over the vertebral column.

Chemical constituents may include:

🟦 terpinyl acetate
🟩 b-caryophyllene
🟨 1.8-cineole

🟧 a-pinene, b-pinene, sabinene
🟪 a-terpineol, terpinen-4-ol

# ROSE OTTO
## Rosa damascena

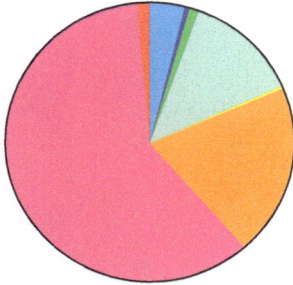

| | | |
|---|---|---|
| ■ | esters | 4.0% |
| ■ | aliphatic aldehydes | 0.5% |
| ■ | ketones | yes |
| ■ | sesquiterpenes | 1.0% |
| ■ | remainder | 12.8% |
| ■ | oxides | 0.3% |
| ■ | monoterpenes | 20.0% |
| ■ | alcohols | 60.0% |
| ■ | phenols, phe. ethers | 1.4% |

## BODY SYSTEMS

**NERVOUS SYSTEM**
■ ■ ■ ■ ■ ■ ■ ■

**ENDOCRINE SYSTEM**
■ ■ ■ ■

**CIRCULATION AND IMMUNE SYSTEM**
■ ■ ■ ■ ■

**SKIN, MUSCLES AND BODY TISSUES**
■ ■ ■ ■ ■ ■ ■

**RESPIRATORY SYSTEM**
■ ■ ■ ■ ■ ■

**DIGESTIVE SYSTEM**
■ ■ ■ ■ ■

**URINARY SYSTEM**
■ ■ ■ ■ ■

**REPRODUCTIVE SYSTEM**
■ ■ ■ ■ ■

## PROPERTIES > USES

aphrodisiac, antispasmodic, balancing, calming, cheering, sedative, tonic > jealousy, increases confidence, Raynaud's disease

regulates, hormone like, stimulates pituarity gland > releases dopamine

bactericidal, decongestant, purifies > stops bleeding, broken veins, tones capillaries, conjunctivitis

antiinflammatory, antiseptic > gingivitis, skin infections, wounds

bactericidal > asthma, bronchitis, coughs, TB

tonic > increases bile production, jaundice, liver, spleen

diuretic >

emmenagogue > frigidity, impotence, pmt

BOTANICAL FAMILY    Rosaceae.

Shrub: distilled petals : sweet heavenly flowery aroma : base note.

Symbol of love and purity. Women's oil to calm and relieve tension and feelings of inadequacy. Scent due to damascenone (only 0.14%).

Chemical constituents may include:

■ citronellyl acetate, geranyl acetate, neryl acetate

■ neral

■ caryophyllene

■ damascenone

■ rose oxide

■ stearoptene, camphene, myrcene, cymene pinenes, ocimene

■ citronellol, geraniol, farnessol, nerol linalool, phenylethyl alcohol

■ methyl eugenol

# ROSEMARY
## Rosmarinus officinalis

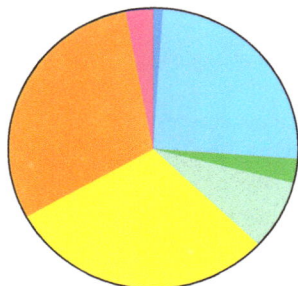

| | | |
|---|---|---|
| 🟦 | esters | 1.0% |
| 🟦 | ketones | 25.0% |
| 🟩 | sesquiterpenes | 3.0% |
| 🟩 | remainder | 8.0% |
| 🟨 | oxides | 30.0% |
| 🟧 | monoterpenes | 30.0% |
| 🟥 | alcohols | 3.0% |

## BODY SYSTEMS

**NERVOUS SYSTEM**
🟦🟦🟩🟨🟧🟥

**ENDOCRINE SYSTEM**
🟦🟨🟧🟥

**CIRCULATION AND IMMUNE SYSTEM**
🟦🟩🟧🟥

**SKIN, MUSCLES AND BODY TISSUES**
🟦🟦🟨🟥

**RESPIRATORY SYSTEM**
🟦🟦🟩🟨🟥

**DIGESTIVE SYSTEM**
🟦🟦🟩🟨🟥

**URINARY SYSTEM**
🟦🟦🟩🟨🟧🟥

**REPRODUCTIVE SYSTEM**
🟦🟦🟩🟨🟧🟥

CAUTIONS
BOTANICAL FAMILY

## PROPERTIES > USES

analgesic, antispasmodic, stimulant, stimulates memory > bed wetting, depression, migraine, Raynaud's disease
stimulates secretions > stimulates central nervous system and bile production
antiviral, astringent, bactericidal, low/high dose lowers/raises blood pressure > arteriosclerosis, circulation, heart
antifungal, antiinflammatory, antiseptic > dissolves swellings and boils, otitis, rheumatism, whooping cough
expectorant, decongestant, mucolytic, stimulant > catarrh, flu
stimulant > constipation, cirrhosis, diarrhoea, flatulence, gall bladder, hepatitis
diuretic > cystitis

emmenagogue > amenorrhoea, candida, scanty periods

Do not use if epilepsy is suspected.
Lamiaceae.

Herb: distilled flowering stalks : strong herbal aroma : middle note.
Name means seadew – Greeks and Romans considered it to be a sacred plant bringing peace and comfort. Can help temporary paralysis and speech problems. Smooth muscle relaxant.
Chemical constituents may include:
🟦 bornyl acetate, fenchyl acetate
🟦 camphor, carvone, thujone, octanone
🟩 caryophyllene, humulene
🟨 1.8-cineole, caryophyllene oxide
🟧 a-pinene, b-pinene, camphene, myrcene, limonene, p-cymene
🟥 terpineol, linalool, borneol, terpinen-4-ol

# ROSEWOOD
### Aniba rosaeodora

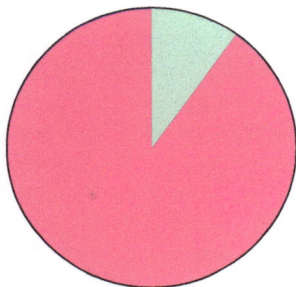

| | | |
|---|---|---|
| ■ | aliphatic aldehydes | yes |
| ■ | ketones | yes |
| ■ | remainder | 10.0% |
| ■ | oxides | yes |
| ■ | monoterpenes | yes |
| ■ | alcohols | 90.0% |

## BODY SYSTEMS

**NERVOUS SYSTEM**
■ ■ ■ ■ ■
**ENDOCRINE SYSTEM**

**CIRCULATION AND IMMUNE SYSTEM**
■ ■ ■ ■
**SKIN, MUSCLES AND BODY TISSUES**
■ ■ ■ ■ ■
**RESPIRATORY SYSTEM**
■ ■ ■ ■
**DIGESTIVE SYSTEM**

**URINARY SYSTEM**

**REPRODUCTIVE SYSTEM**
■ ■ ■

BOTANICAL FAMILY

## PROPERTIES > USES

analgesic, aphrodisiac, stimulant, tonic > clears mind, depression

antiviral, bactericidal, immune system tonic > chronic conditions
antifungal, antiseptic, deodorant, insecticide > skin tonic and healer
antiseptic > bronchopneumonia, ticklish coughs

antifungal > candida

Lauraceae: the gentle member of this family which is generally powerful and stimulating.

Tree: distilled heartwood : sweet floral woody aroma : middle note.
Brazilian exploitation of the forests to produce oil has now been restricted and replanting programmes are in place.

Chemical constituents may include:

■ citronellal
■ 1.8-cineole, linalool oxide
■ a-terpinene, limonene, b-pinene
■ linalool, geraniol, nerol, a-terpineol

# SAGE COMMON
## Salvia officinalis

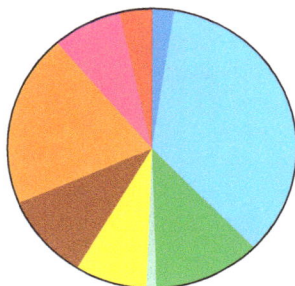

| | | |
|---|---|---|
| 🟦 | esters | 2.5% |
| 🟦 | aliphatic aldehydes | yes |
| 🟦 | ketones | 35.0% |
| 🟩 | sesquiterpenes | 12.0% |
| 🟩 | lactones and coumarins | yes |
| ⬜ | remainder | 1.0% |
| 🟨 | oxides | 8.0% |
| 🟫 | aromatic aldehydes | 10.0% |
| 🟧 | monoterpenes | 20.0% |
| 🟪 | alcohols | 8.0% |
| 🟧 | phenols, phe. ethers | 3.5% |

## BODY SYSTEMS

NERVOUS SYSTEM
🟦🟦🟦🟩🟩🟨🟫🟧🟪🟧

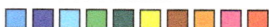

ENDOCRINE SYSTEM
🟦🟧

CIRCULATION AND IMMUNE SYSTEM
🟦🟦🟦🟩🟩🟨🟫🟧🟪🟧

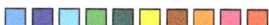

SKIN, MUSCLES AND BODY TISSUES
🟦🟦🟦🟩🟩🟨🟫🟧🟪🟧

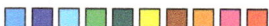

RESPIRATORY SYSTEM
🟦🟦🟦🟩🟩🟨🟫🟧🟪🟧

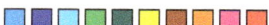

DIGESTIVE SYSTEM
🟦🟦🟨🟫🟧

URINARY SYSTEM
🟦🟦🟨🟫🟧

REPRODUCTIVE SYSTEM
🟦🟦🟦🟩🟩🟨🟫🟧🟪🟧

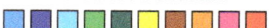

CAUTIONS

BOTANICAL FAMILY

## PROPERTIES > USES

analgesic, antispasmodic, tonic > eases trembling, meningitis, neuritis, palsy
stops milk production, stimulates secretions > bile

antiviral, bactericidal, decongestant, purifies, raises blood pressure, tonic > balances circulation
antifungal, antiseptic > cellulite, malignancies, oedema, psoriasis, rheumatoid arthritis, toothache, ulcers, wounds
expectorant, mucolytic > bronchitis, catarrh, flu

stimulant, tonic > bile, liver, pancreas

diuretic >

abortive, emmenagogue > candida, genital herpes, hot flushes, leucorrhoea, thrush

Avoid in pregnancy. Do not use with young children or epileptics. Not recommended by some practitioners. Lamiaceae.

Herb: distilled flowering herb : sharp herbal aroma : top note. Hailed as a miracle plant by the Romans – 'salvare' means to heal, to save. Used as a nerve tonic through the middle ages. Chemical constituents may include:

🟦 bornyl acetate, linalyl acetate
🟦 hexanal
🟦 a-thujone, b-thujone, camphor, fenchone
🟩 caryophyllene, humulene, cadinene

🟨 1.8-cineole, caryophyllene oxide
🟧 a-pinene, b-pinene, phellandrene, camphene, myrcene, limonene, p-cymene
🟪 borneol, viridiflorol, linalool, terpinen-4-ol
🟧 methyl chavicol (estragole), thymol

# SAGE SPANISH
## Salvia lavendulaefolia

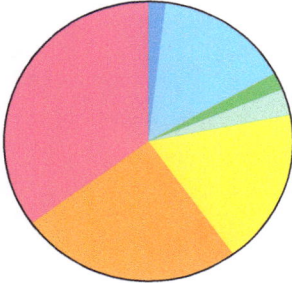

| | | |
|---|---|---|
| ■ | esters | 2.0% |
| ■ | ketones | 15.0% |
| ■ | sesquiterpenes | 2.0% |
| ■ | remainder | 3.0% |
| ■ | oxides | 18.0% |
| ■ | acids | yes |
| ■ | monoterpenes | 25.0% |
| ■ | alcohols | 35.0% |

## BODY SYSTEMS

NERVOUS SYSTEM
■ ■ ■ ■ ■

ENDOCRINE SYSTEM
■ ■ ■

CIRCULATION AND IMMUNE SYSTEM
■ ■ ■ ■

SKIN, MUSCLES AND BODY TISSUES
■ ■ ■ ■ ■ ■

RESPIRATORY SYSTEM
■ ■ ■ ■

DIGESTIVE SYSTEM
■ ■ ■ ■

URINARY SYSTEM

REPRODUCTIVE SYSTEM
■ ■ ■ ■ ■

CAUTIONS

BOTANICAL FAMILY

## PROPERTIES > USES

antispasmodic, tonic > headaches, nervous exhaustion, neuralgia

lowers fever, regulates sebum production, reduces sweating > stimulates liver and adrenal cortex

astringent, lowers blood pressure > circulation, purifies blood

antiinflammatory, antiseptic > acne, arthritis, eczema, fluid retention, gingivitis, hair loss, rheumatism, wounds

decongestant, expectorant > asthma, catarrh, coughs, flu, rhinitis, sinusitis

stimulant > congested liver, jaundice

emmenagogue > amenorrhoea, painful periods

Avoid in pregnancy. Use in moderation.

Lamiaceae.

Herb: distilled flowering herb : sage like lavender aroma : top note.
In Spain considered a 'cure all'. Some chemotypes have much higher percentages of camphor present hence the need for caution.

Chemical constituents may include:
■ linalyl acetate, bornyl acetate, sabinyl acetate, terpinyl acetate
■ camphor
■ caryophyllene, humulene, bergaptene

■ 1.8-cineole
■ a-pinene, b-pinene, sabinene, myrcene, limonene, p-cymene, camphene
■ linalool, a-terpineol, borneol, sabinol, geraniol

# SANDALWOOD
## Santalum album

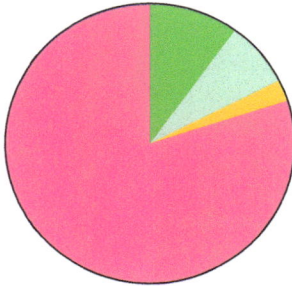

| | | |
|---|---|---|
| ■ | aliphatic aldehydes | yes |
| ■ | ketones | yes |
| ■ | sesquiterpenes | 10.0% |
| ■ | lactones and coumarins | yes |
| ■ | remainder | 7.5% |
| ■ | acids | 2.5% |
| ■ | monoterpenes | yes |
| ■ | alcohols | 80.0% |
| ■ | phenols, phe. ethers | yes |

BODY SYSTEMS

PROPERTIES > USES

NERVOUS SYSTEM
■ ■ ■ ■ ■

aphrodisiac, calming, sedative, tonic > bereavement, impotence, neuralgia, sciatica

ENDOCRINE SYSTEM
■ ■

promotes vaginal secretions >

CIRCULATION AND IMMUNE SYSTEM
■ ■ ■ ■ ■

astringent, bactericidal, decongestant > heart regulation, varicose veins

SKIN, MUSCLES AND BODY TISSUES
■ ■ ■ ■ ■ ■ ■

antiinflammatory, antiseptic > aging skin, dry ezcema, itching, haemorrhoids, lumbago

RESPIRATORY SYSTEM
■ ■ ■ ■ ■ ■ ■

calming > catarrh, eases coughs

DIGESTIVE SYSTEM
■ ■ ■ ■

calming > diarrhoea

URINARY SYSTEM
■ ■ ■ ■ ■

diuretic > cystitis, kidney

REPRODUCTIVE SYSTEM
■ ■ ■ ■ ■ ■

antiseptic > gonorrhoea

BOTANICAL FAMILY

Santalaceae.

Tree: distilled heartwood : musty lingering aroma : base note.
Brings peaceful feelings. Comfort to the dying. Used in incenses and meditation.

Chemical constituents may include:

■ santalone
■ santalenes, curcumenes, farnesene
■ limonene

■ nortricloekasantalic acid
■ santalols, tricloekasantalol, borneol

# SAVORY SUMMER
## Satureja hortensis

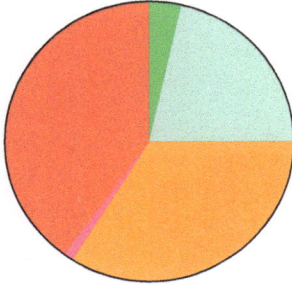

| | | |
|---|---|---|
| ☐ | ketones | yes |
| ☐ | sesquiterpenes | 3.5% |
| ☐ | remainder | 21.5% |
| ☐ | oxides | yes |
| ☐ | acids | yes |
| ☐ | aromatic aldehydes | yes |
| ☐ | monoterpenes | 34.0% |
| ☐ | alcohols | 1.0% |
| ☐ | phenols, phe. ethers | 40.0% |

## BODY SYSTEMS

**NERVOUS SYSTEM**

**ENDOCRINE SYSTEM**

**CIRCULATION AND IMMUNE SYSTEM**

**SKIN, MUSCLES AND BODY TISSUES**

**RESPIRATORY SYSTEM**

**DIGESTIVE SYSTEM**

**URINARY SYSTEM**

**REPRODUCTIVE SYSTEM**

## PROPERTIES > USES

aphrodisiac, general tonic >

stimulates secretions > bile

antiviral, astringent, strongly bactericidal, tonic > cardiac

antifungal, air antiseptic, irritant, parasiticide, vulnerary > any infected location

expectorant > mucous membrane irritant

stimulant > liver, facilitates elimination, flatulence

sexual tonic >

CAUTIONS — Avoid during pregnancy. Not recommended for use by some practitioners due to high phenol content. Do not use directly onto skin.

BOTANICAL FAMILY — Lamiaceae.

Herb: distilled whole dried herb : strong thyme like aroma : top note.
Closely related to the thymes. Popular for cookery, peppery flavour. Therapeutic tea for digestion, respiratory and menstrual problems.

Chemical constituents may include:

☐ camphor
☐ b-caryophyllene, bisabolene, cadinene
☐ damascenone
☐ 1.8-cineole
☐ piperonal
☐ a-terpinene, g-terpinene, p-cymene, myrcene, pinenes, limonene, phellandrene
☐ linalool, borneol, terpineol, terpinen-4-ol
☐ thymol, eugenol, carvacrol

# SAVORY WINTER
## Satureja montana

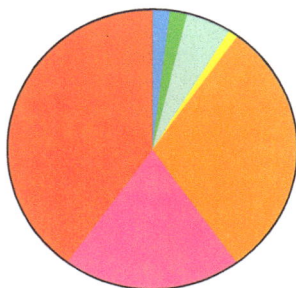

| | | |
|---|---|---|
| 🟦 | esters | 2.0% |
| ⬜ | ketones | yes |
| 🟩 | sesquiterpenes | 2.0% |
| 🟢 | remainder | 5.0% |
| 🟨 | oxides | 1.0% |
| 🟨 | acids | yes |
| 🟧 | monoterpenes | 30.0% |
| 🟥 | alcohols | 20.0% |
| 🟧 | phenols, phe. ethers | 40.0% |

## BODY SYSTEMS

**NERVOUS SYSTEM**

**ENDOCRINE SYSTEM**

**CIRCULATION AND IMMUNE SYSTEM**

**SKIN, MUSCLES AND BODY TISSUES**

**RESPIRATORY SYSTEM**

**DIGESTIVE SYSTEM**

**URINARY SYSTEM**

**REPRODUCTIVE SYSTEM**

CAUTIONS

BOTANICAL FAMILY

Herb: distilled whole dried herb : herby medicinal aroma : top note.
Highly antiseptic properties.
Chemical constituents may include:

🟦 linalyl acetate, terpinyl acetate, geranyl acetate
⬜ camphor
🟩 b-caryophyllene, humulene
🟢 damascenone

🟨 1.8-cineole, caryophyllene oxide
🟧 a-terpinene, g-terpinene, p-cymene, pinenes limonene
🟥 linalool, borneol, a-terpineol, thujanols
🟧 carvacrol, thymol, eugenol

## PROPERTIES > USES

general tonic, mental stimulant, neurotonic > depression, nervous exhaustion

antiviral, strongly bactericidal, raises blood pressure, immune system tonic > circulation
antifungal, strongly antiseptic, irritant > abscesses, fungal infection of mouth, impetigo, rheumatoid arthritis
bactericidal > bronchitis, coughs, malaria, TB

bactericidal > colic, colitis, diarrhoea, enteritis, flatulence, intestinal spasm
duretic > cystitis, prostate, renal TB

antifungal > candida

Avoid in pregnancy. Not recommended for use by some practitioners due to its high phenol content. Do not use directly onto skin.
Lamiaceae.

80

# SPRUCE CANADIAN BLACK

## Picea mariana nigra

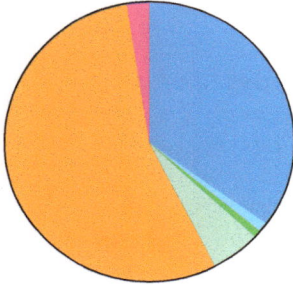

| | | |
|---|---|---|
| ■ | esters | 35.0% |
| ■ | ketones | 1.0% |
| ■ | sesquiterpenes | 1.0% |
| ■ | remainder | 5.5% |
| ■ | monoterpenes | 55.0% |
| ■ | alcohols | 2.5% |

### BODY SYSTEMS

**NERVOUS SYSTEM**
■ ■ ■ ■

**ENDOCRINE SYSTEM**
■ ■

**CIRCULATION AND IMMUNE SYSTEM**
■ ■ ■

**SKIN, MUSCLES AND BODY TISSUES**
■ ■ ■ ■ ■

**RESPIRATORY SYSTEM**
■ ■ ■ ■ ■

**DIGESTIVE SYSTEM**

**URINARY SYSTEM**

**REPRODUCTIVE SYSTEM**
■ ■ ■

BOTANICAL FAMILY

### PROPERTIES > USES

antispasmodic, tonic > revitalising

cortisone like, hormone like > overactive thyroid, ovaries, thymus gland

bactericidal, immune system tonic >

antifungal, antiinflammatory, air antiseptic, tonic > acne, eczema, rheumatism

bactericidal > bronchitis

antifungal > candida

Pinaceae: this family is generally highly antiseptic and aids respiratory problems.

Tree: distilled young branches and leaves : pleasant pine needle aroma : middle note. Often added to pine and cedar oils.

Chemical constituents may include:

■ bornyl acetate
■ camphor
■ longifolene, longicyclene, cadinene

■ tricyclene, a-pinene, d-carene, camphene
■ borneol, longiborneol

# SPRUCE HEMLOCK
## Tsuga canadensis

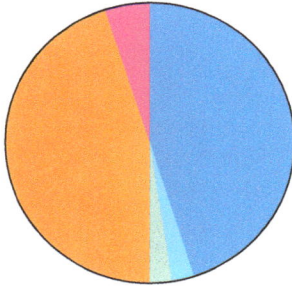

| | | |
|---|---|---|
| | esters | 45.0% |
| | aliphatic aldehydes | yes |
| | ketones | 2.5% |
| | sesquiterpenes | yes |
| | remainder | 2.5% |
| | monoterpenes | 45.0% |
| | alcohols | 5.0% |

BODY SYSTEMS

NERVOUS SYSTEM

ENDOCRINE SYSTEM

CIRCULATION AND IMMUNE SYSTEM

SKIN, MUSCLES AND BODY TISSUES

RESPIRATORY SYSTEM

DIGESTIVE SYSTEM

URINARY SYSTEM

REPRODUCTIVE SYSTEM

BOTANICAL FAMILY

PROPERTIES > USES

calming, stimulant > anxiety, stress

bactericidal, stems bleeding, lymph system tonic > lymph circulation

antiseptic > aches and pains, rheumatism

expectorant > asthma, bronchitis, coughs, weakness

diuretic >

Pinaceae: this family is generally highly antiseptic and aids respiratory problems.

Tree: distilled needles and twigs : fresh fruity sweet aroma : middle note.
Widely used for veterinary linaments and for room sprays.

Chemical constituents may include:

bornyl acetate
thujone
cadinene

pinenes, limonene, tricyclene, camphene, myrcene, phellandrene, dipentene
borneol

# TAGETES
## Tagetes glandulifera

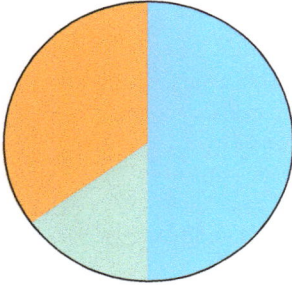

| | | |
|---|---|---|
| ■ | aliphatic aldehydes | yes |
| □ | ketones | 50.0% |
| ■ | lactones and coumarins | yes |
| □ | remainder | 15.0% |
| □ | acids | yes |
| ■ | aromatic aldehydes | yes |
| ■ | monoterpenes | 35.0% |
| ■ | alcohols | yes |

## BODY SYSTEMS

**NERVOUS SYSTEM**
■ ■ □ ■ ■
**ENDOCRINE SYSTEM**

**CIRCULATION AND IMMUNE SYSTEM**
■ ■ ■ ■ ■
**SKIN, MUSCLES AND BODY TISSUES**
■ ■ □ ■ ■ ■

**RESPIRATORY SYSTEM**
□ ■ ■ ■
**DIGESTIVE SYSTEM**

**URINARY SYSTEM**

**REPRODUCTIVE SYSTEM**
□

CAUTIONS

BOTANICAL FAMILY

## PROPERTIES > USES

antispasmodic, sedative > clears mind, firmer hold on emotions, relieves tension, sharpens senses

bactericidal, lowers blood pressure >

antifungal, antiinflammatory, antiseptic, cell generator, insecticide > athlete's foot, bunions, callouses, corns, flies, ear infections, maggots, mosquitoes
decongestant > affinity to respiratory system, bronchial dilator, coughs

emmenagogue >

Powerful oil use with care, check for skin irritation.

Compositae: this family is generally soothing especially for the skin and digestion.

Plant: distilled after the full flowering stage : strong marigold aroma : top note.
Often planted among vegetables to deter pests. Used extensively in French perfumes.

Chemical constituents may include:

■ citral
□ tagetone, tagetenones, carvone
□ valeric acid

■ salicylaldehyde
□ pinenes, limonene, ocimene, myrcene, camphene
■ linalool

# TARRAGON
## Artemisia dracunculus

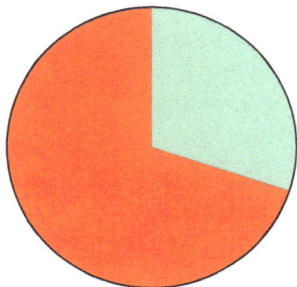

| | | |
|---|---|---|
| ☐ | ketones | yes |
| ☐ | lactones and coumarins | 0.1% |
| ☐ | remainder | 29.9% |
| ☐ | oxides | yes |
| ☐ | monoterpenes | yes |
| ☐ | alcohols | yes |
| ☐ | phenols, phe. ethers | 70.0% |

## BODY SYSTEMS

**NERVOUS SYSTEM**
☐☐☐☐☐☐

**ENDOCRINE SYSTEM**
☐☐☐

**CIRCULATION AND IMMUNE SYSTEM**
☐☐☐☐☐☐

**SKIN, MUSCLES AND BODY TISSUES**
☐☐☐☐☐☐

**RESPIRATORY SYSTEM**
☐☐☐☐☐

**DIGESTIVE SYSTEM**
☐☐☐☐☐☐

**URINARY SYSTEM**
☐☐☐☐☐

**REPRODUCTIVE SYSTEM**
☐☐☐☐

CAUTIONS

BOTANICAL FAMILY

## PROPERTIES > USES

antispasmodic, hypnotic, neuromuscular tonic, stimulant > allergies, neuralgia, pmt, sciatica
balances menstrual cycle, stimulates secretion > bile
antiviral, bactericidal, decongestant, purifies > chronic conditions
antiinflammatory, antiseptic > arthritis (clears uric acid), rheumatism, weeping wounds
decongestant > hiccoughs

stimulates appetite > anorexia, bile secretion, digestion heavy fats, inflamed intestines, laxative, spasms, worms
diuretic > cleanses kidneys

emmenagogue > amenorrhoea, menstrual, painful periods, pmt

Avoid in pregnancy, use with care due to large amount of phenols present.
Compositae: this family is generally soothing especially for the skin and digestion.

Herb: distilled leaves : spicy aniseed like aroma : top note. Very popular culinary herb rich in vitamins A and C. Has been used to treat snake and dog bites.

Chemical constituents may include:
☐ thujone
☐ aesculetin, methyl oxycoumarin, herniarine
☐ 1.8-cineole
☐ ocimene, phellandrene
☐ nerol
☐ methyl chavicol (estragole), anethole

# TEATREE
## Melaleuca alternifolia

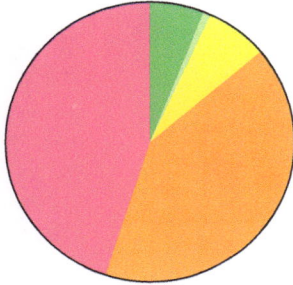

| | | |
|---|---|---|
| 🟩 | sesquiterpenes | 6.0% |
| 🟦 | remainder | 1.0% |
| 🟨 | oxides | 7.0% |
| 🟧 | acids | yes |
| 🟧 | monoterpenes | 41.0% |
| 🟥 | alcohols | 45.0% |

## BODY SYSTEMS

**NERVOUS SYSTEM**
🟩⬜🟧🟥

**ENDOCRINE SYSTEM**
🟦🟥

**CIRCULATION AND IMMUNE SYSTEM**
🟩⬜🟨🟧🟥

**SKIN, MUSCLES AND BODY TISSUES**
🟩🟦🟨⬜🟧🟥

**RESPIRATORY SYSTEM**
🟩⬜🟧🟥

**DIGESTIVE SYSTEM**
🟩🟧🟥

**URINARY SYSTEM**
🟩🟧🟥

**REPRODUCTIVE SYSTEM**
🟨🟧🟥

## BOTANICAL FAMILY

## PROPERTIES > USES

analgesic, neurotonic > depression, hysteria, shock

causes sweating >

antiviral, strongly bactericidal, decongestant, immune system tonic, heart tonic > varicose veins
antifungal, antiinflammatory, strongly antiseptic, parasiticide > athlete's foot, bites, boils, burns, radiography burns, cold sores, itching, mouth ulcers, ringworm, spots, sweaty feet, wounds
bactericidal > asthma, bronchitis, catarrh, TB, whooping cough
antiseptic > haemorrhoids, mouth infections

bactericidal > cystitis

antifungal > candida, congested ovaries, thrush

Myrtaceae: this family is generally stimulating and good for the respiratory system.

Shrub: distilled leaves : pungent sanitary aroma : top note.
Extensively used in aboriginal medicine, wide spread current use including surgical and dental practices. Strong antifungal agent.

Chemical constituents may include:
🟩 aromadendrene, viridiflorene, cadinene, caryophyllene
🟨 1.8-cineole, 1.4-cineole
🟧 a-pinene, a-terpinene, g-terpinene, p-cymene, limonene, terpinolene, myrcene
🟥 terpinen-4-ol, a-terpineol, globulol, viridiflorol

# THUJA WHITE CEDAR
## Thuja occidentalis

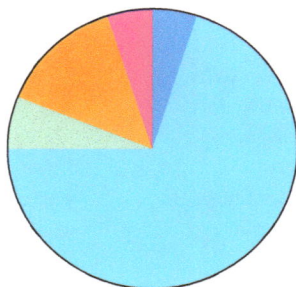

| | | |
|---|---|---|
| | esters | 5.0% |
| | ketones | 70.0% |
| | sesquiterpenes | yes |
| | remainder | 6.0% |
| | acids | yes |
| | monoterpenes | 14.0% |
| | alcohols | 5.0% |

## BODY SYSTEMS

**NERVOUS SYSTEM**

**ENDOCRINE SYSTEM**

**CIRCULATION AND IMMUNE SYSTEM**

**SKIN, MUSCLES AND BODY TISSUES**

**RESPIRATORY SYSTEM**

**DIGESTIVE SYSTEM**

**URINARY SYSTEM**

**REPRODUCTIVE SYSTEM**

CAUTIONS

BOTANICAL FAMILY

## PROPERTIES > USES

stimulant >

astringent, heart tonic >

stimulant > insect repellent, rheumatism, warts

expectorant >

parasiticide, vermifuge > poison

diuretic >

abortive, stimulant >

Not recommended for use except in exceptional circumstances.

Cupressaceae: this family generally aids nervous tension, rheumatism and cellulite.

Tree: distilled leaves twigs and bark : sharp camphor like aroma : top note.
Used as incense by ancient civilisations. Twigs are currently in the British Herbal Pharmacoepia for cardiac weakness, bronchitis and warts.

Chemical constituents may include:
- bornyl acetate
- thujone, camphor, fenchone, piperitone, isothujone
- pinene, sabinene
- terpinen-4-ol, occidentalol, occidol

# THYME COMMON RED OR WHITE
## Thymus vulgaris thymoliferum

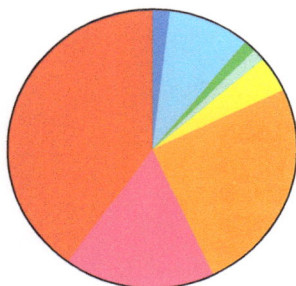

| | | |
|---|---|---|
| 🟦 | esters | 2.0% |
| 🟦 | ketones | 9.0% |
| 🟩 | sesquiterpenes | 1.5% |
| 🟩 | remainder | 1.5% |
| 🟨 | oxides | 4.0% |
| 🟨 | acids | yes |
| 🟧 | monoterpenes | 25.0% |
| 🟥 | alcohols | 17.0% |
| 🟥 | phenols, phe. ethers | 40.0% |

## BODY SYSTEMS

**NERVOUS SYSTEM**

**ENDOCRINE SYSTEM**

**CIRCULATION AND IMMUNE SYSTEM**

**SKIN, MUSCLES AND BODY TISSUES**

**RESPIRATORY SYSTEM**

**DIGESTIVE SYSTEM**

**URINARY SYSTEM**

**REPRODUCTIVE SYSTEM**

CAUTIONS
BOTANICAL FAMILY

## PROPERTIES > USES

antispasmodic, general and neurotonic, mental sexual tonic, stimulant > depression, stress
causes sweating > stimulates white corpuscles

bactericidal, raises blood pressure, capillary stimulant > anaemia, circulation
antioxidant, antiseptic, parasiticide > acne, arthritis, boils, carbuncles, hair loss, rheumatism, wounds
expectorant > anxiety, asthma, bronchial secretions

stimulant > flatulence, sluggish digestion, worms

diuretic > cystitis

mucolytic > assists childbirth, helps to expel afterbirth, leucorrhoea

Avoid in cases of pregnancy or high blood pressure.
Lamiaceae.

Herb: distilled fresh or part dried leaves and flowering tops : strong herby aroma : top note. Composition of thyme oils is complex to identify. Strongly bactericidal. Red Thyme and White Thyme have high phenol content as shown above. White Thyme is a refined distillation of Red Thyme. Sweet Thyme is a very different oil and is shown on page 88. Chemical constituents may include:

🟦 linalyl acetate, terpinyl acetate
🟦 camphor, thujone
🟩 b-caryophyllene
🟨 1.8-cineole, linalool oxide
🟧 p-cymene, g-terpinene, a-pinene, camphene, myrcene, limonene, terpinolene
🟥 borneol, linalool, terpinen-4-ol
🟥 thymol, carvacrol

87

# THYME COMMON SWEET

## Thymus vulgaris linaloliferum or geranioliferum

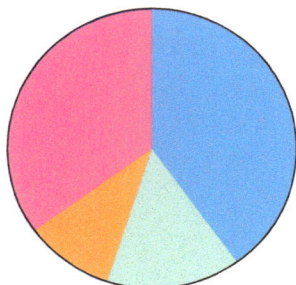

| | | |
|---|---|---|
| 🟦 | esters | 40.0% |
| 🟦 | ketones | yes |
| 🟩 | sesquiterpenes | yes |
| 🟩 | remainder | 15.0% |
| 🟨 | oxides | yes |
| 🟧 | acids | yes |
| 🟧 | monoterpenes | 10.0% |
| 🟪 | alcohols | 35.0% |
| 🟥 | phenols, phe. ethers | yes |

## BODY SYSTEMS

**NERVOUS SYSTEM**

**ENDOCRINE SYSTEM**

**CIRCULATION AND IMMUNE SYSTEM**

**SKIN, MUSCLES AND BODY TISSUES**

**RESPIRATORY SYSTEM**

**DIGESTIVE SYSTEM**

**URINARY SYSTEM**

**REPRODUCTIVE SYSTEM**

## PROPERTIES > USES

antispasmodic > fatigue

stimulates secretions > bile

antiviral > heart stimulant

antioxidant, antifungal, antiinflammatory,
antiseptic > acne, dry and wet eczema, muscular
rheumatism, psoriasis, verrucas
antiseptic > bronchitis, bronchial spasm, sinusitis,
sore throat, tonsillitis, TB
antiviral > colitis, diarrhoea, liver, viral enteritis

antiseptic > cystitis, urethritis

antifungal, uterine tonic > assists childbirth,
candida, vaginitis

BOTANICAL FAMILY    Lamiaceae.

Herb: distilled fresh or part dried leaves and flowering tops : sweet lemon aroma : top note.
Much safer to use than thymus vulgaris thymoliferum (red or white thyme).

Chemical constituents may include:

🟦 linalyl acetate, geranyl acetate    🟪 linalool or geraniol

# THYME MOROCCAN
## Thymus satureioides

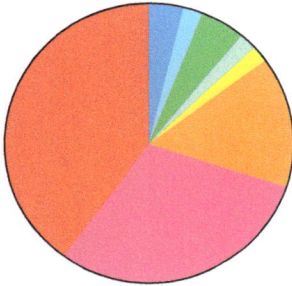

| | | |
|---|---|---|
| 🟦 | esters | 4.0% |
| 🟪 | aliphatic aldehydes | yes |
| 🟦 | ketones | 2.0% |
| 🟩 | sesquiterpenes | 5.0% |
| 🟩 | remainder | 2.0% |
| 🟨 | oxides | 2.0% |
| 🟨 | acids | yes |
| 🟧 | monoterpenes | 15.0% |
| 🟥 | alcohols | 30.0% |
| 🟧 | phenols, phe. ethers | 40.0% |

## BODY SYSTEMS

**NERVOUS SYSTEM**
🟦🟪🟦🟨🟨🟧🟥🟧

**ENDOCRINE SYSTEM**
🟦🟧

**CIRCULATION AND IMMUNE SYSTEM**
🟩🟨🟥🟧

**SKIN, MUSCLES AND BODY TISSUES**
🟦🟪🟦🟩🟨🟨🟧🟥🟧

**RESPIRATORY SYSTEM**
🟦🟩🟨🟥🟧

**DIGESTIVE SYSTEM**
🟦🟧

**URINARY SYSTEM**
🟦🟪🟦🟩🟨🟨🟥🟧

**REPRODUCTIVE SYSTEM**
🟨🟨🟥🟧

## PROPERTIES > USES

sexual tonic, stimulant, neurotonic > debility, general fatigue
stimulates secretions > gall bladder, gastric, liver

bactericidal, immune system tonic >

antiinflammatory, antiseptic, possible irritant > acne, arthritis, chronic sinusitis, tonsillitis
bactericidal > TB

secretions > gall bladder, gall stones, liver

bactericidal > cystitis

uterine tonic >

**BOTANICAL FAMILY**    Lamiaceae.

Herb: distilled flowering tops : herby aroma : top note.
Similar properties to thymus vulgaris thymoliferum (red or white thyme).

Chemical constituents may include:

🟦 bornyl acetate, linalyl acetate
🟦 dihydrocarvone, verbenone, camphor
🟩 caryophyllene, cadinene, copaene, bourbonene, humulene

🟨 1.8-cineole, caryophyllene oxide, linalool oxide
🟧 a-pinene, g-terpinene, p-cymene, camphene
🟥 borneol, terpineol, terpinen-4-ol, linalool
🟧 methyl chavicol (estragole), thymol, carvacrol

# VETIVER
## Vetiveria zizanoides

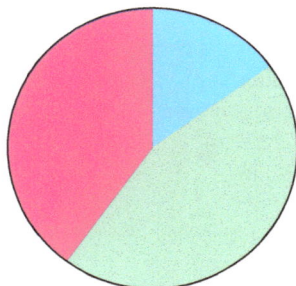

| | | |
|---|---|---|
| ■ | esters | yes |
| ■ | ketones | 15.0% |
| ■ | sesquiterpenes | yes |
| ☐ | remainder | 45.0% |
| ■ | acids | yes |
| ■ | alcohols | 40.0% |

## BODY SYSTEMS

NERVOUS SYSTEM
■ ■ ■ ■

ENDOCRINE SYSTEM
■ ■ ■ ■

CIRCULATION AND IMMUNE SYSTEM
■ ■ ■

SKIN, MUSCLES AND BODY TISSUES
■ ■ ■ ■ ■

RESPIRATORY SYSTEM

DIGESTIVE SYSTEM
■ ■

URINARY SYSTEM

REPRODUCTIVE SYSTEM
■ ■ ■

BOTANICAL FAMILY

## PROPERTIES > USES

aphrodisiac, calming, sedative, tonic > dentist's visit, over sensitivity, protective shield, stress, tension
stimulant to glands > promotes bleeding, promotes pancreas secretions
immune system tonic, stimulates blood flow > coronary arteries, veins
antiseptic > aches and pains, acne, arthritis, rheumatism

stimulant > congested liver, pancreas

emmenagogue > amenorrhoea, scanty periods

Gramineae.

Grass: distilled roots : earthy woody aroma : base note.
Known as the oil of tranquillity. The grass is called 'kuskus' and is used to make awnings, sunshades and blinds. Beautiful aroma when dampened.

Chemical constituents may include:

| | | |
|---|---|---|
| ■ vetiverol acetate | ☐ furfural |
| ■ vetiverone | ■ vetivenic acid, benzoic acid, palmitic acid |
| ■ vetivene, vetivazulene | ■ vetiverol |

# YARROW
## Achillea millefolium

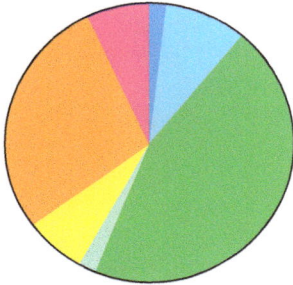

| | | |
|---|---|---|
| ■ | esters | 2.0% |
| ■ | ketones | 9.0% |
| ■ | sesquiterpenes | 45.0% |
| ■ | lactones and coumarins | yes |
| ■ | remainder | 2.0% |
| ■ | oxides | 7.0% |
| ■ | acids | yes |
| ■ | monoterpenes | 28.0% |
| ■ | alcohols | 7.0% |
| ■ | phenols, phe. ethers | yes |

## BODY SYSTEMS

NERVOUS SYSTEM

ENDOCRINE SYSTEM

CIRCULATION AND IMMUNE SYSTEM

SKIN, MUSCLES AND BODY TISSUES

RESPIRATORY SYSTEM

DIGESTIVE SYSTEM

URINARY SYSTEM

REPRODUCTIVE SYSTEM

CAUTIONS

BOTANICAL FAMILY

## PROPERTIES > USES

antispasmodic, tonic > neuralgia, stress

causes sweating, hormone like, temperature reducing, stimulates secretions > bile, good woman's oil

acts on the bone marrow stimulates blood renewal, astringent, lowers blood pressure, decongestant > varicose veins

antiinflammatory, antiseptic, cell generator > baldness, back ache, ulcers, wounds

antiseptic > catarrh

stimulant > diarrhoea

balances urine flow and urine retention, diuretic > bed wetting, cystitis, kidney scars

abortive, emmenagogue > fibroids, ovaries, period problems, prolapse

Avoid in pregnancy and with young children powerful oil.

Compositae: this family is generally soothing especially for the skin and digestion.

Plant: distilled flowering heads : sweet spicy camphorous aroma : middle note.
Used in Scotland to ward off evil spirits. Considered an 'all healing' plant.
Chemical constituents may include:

■ bornyl acetate
■ isoartemisia, camphor, thujone
■ chamazulene, caryophyllene, germacrene, dihydroazulene
■ achilline

■ 1.8-cineole, caryophyllene oxide
■ limonene, a-pinene, b-pinene, sabinene, camphene, myrcene
■ borneol, terpinen-4-ol, cadinol
■ eugenol

# YLANG YLANG
## Cananga odorata

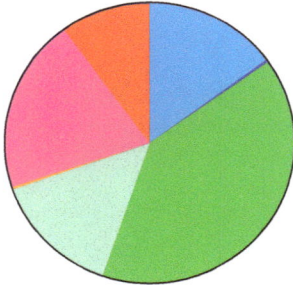

| | | |
|---|---|---|
| ■ | esters | 15.0% |
| ■ | aliphatic aldehydes | 0.1% |
| ■ | ketones | 0.1% |
| ■ | sesquiterpenes | 40.0% |
| ■ | remainder | 14.4% |
| ■ | acids | yes |
| ■ | monoterpenes | 0.4% |
| ■ | alcohols | 20.0% |
| ■ | phenols, phe. ethers | 10.0% |

## BODY SYSTEMS

NERVOUS SYSTEM
■ ■ ■ ■ ■ ■ ■

ENDOCRINE SYSTEM
■ ■ ■ ■ ■

CIRCULATION AND IMMUNE SYSTEM
■ ■ ■ ■ ■ ■

SKIN, MUSCLES AND BODY TISSUES
■ ■ ■ ■ ■ ■

RESPIRATORY SYSTEM
■ ■ ■ ■

DIGESTIVE SYSTEM
■ ■ ■ ■ ■ ■

URINARY SYSTEM

REPRODUCTIVE SYSTEM
■ ■ ■ ■ ■ ■ ■

CAUTIONS

BOTANICAL FAMILY

## PROPERTIES > USES

aphrodisiac, antispasmodic, balancing, calming, sedative, tonic > anxiety, depression, fear, panic, shock
regulates adrenaline flow >

lowers blood pressure, balances sebum production > slows heart beat

antiseptic > possible skin irritation, stimulates hair growth

calming > slows breathing pace

stimulates secretions > diabetes, gastric, intestinal infections

stimulates ovaries and testicles > frigidity, impotence

Use with care can cause headaches and nausea.

Annonaceae.

Small tree: distilled flowers : sweet heavy exotic aroma : base note.
In Indonesia wedding beds are strewn with the flower petals. Used extensively in perfumes.

Chemical constituents may include:

■ methyl benzoate, methyl salicylate, benzyl acetate, benzyl benzoate, geranyl acetate
■ b-caryophyllene, cadinene, farnesene, germacrene, humulene
■ pinenes
■ farnesol, geraniol, linalool, benzyl alcohol
■ methyl eugenol, eugenol, safrole, p-cresyl methyl ether

# Part Two

---

# 50 Therapeutic Blends for 50 Common Ailments

# Acne

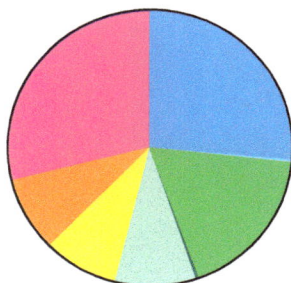

| | | |
|---|---|---|
| ■ | esters | 26.2% |
| ■ | aliphatic aldehydes | trace |
| ■ | ketones | 0.1% |
| ■ | sesquiterpenes | 18.5% |
| ■ | lactones & coumarins | 0.2% |
| ■ | remainder | 9.0% |
| ■ | oxides | 8.6% |
| ■ | acids | trace |
| ■ | aromatic aldehydes | trace |
| ■ | monoterpenes | 8.0% |
| ■ | alcohols | 29.4% |
| ■ | phenols, phe. ethers | trace |

**CCP of BLEND RECIPE**

*Orange Petitgrain* (citrus aurantium amara)

*Chamomile Maroc* (ormenis multicaulis)

*Niaouli* (melaleuca viridiflora)

*Cedar Virginian Red* (juniperus virginiana)

*Orange Petitgrain* is a strongly bactericidal and is also a calming and cheering oil. It recommended to treat infected acne. The aroma is woody and floral.

*Chamomile Maroc* is an effective antiseptic, decongestant and bactericidal. It is recommended for eczema, dry cracked skin, infected pus and acne.

*Niaouli* is highly antiseptic and tones and heals skin conditions including acne, boils, spots and ulcers.

*Cedar Virginian Red* helps to tone oily skin. Treats acne, eczema and dandruff.

*Chemical constituents to be found in the blend may include:*

■ linalyl acetate, geranyl acetate, neryl acetate, bornyl acetate, bornyl butyrate
■ β-caryophyllene, bisabolene, cedrene, germacrene, thujopsene
■ 1.8-cineole
■ α-pinene, β-pinene, myrcene, limonene
■ linalool, geraniol, α-terpineol, santolina alcohol, yomogi alcohol, artemisia alcohol, viridiflorol, cedrol, globulol, widdrol, γ-eudesmol.

## BLEND

| | |
|---|---|
| 18 drops | *Orange Petitgrain* |
| 6 drops | *Chamomile Maroc* |
| 6 drops | *Niaouli* |
| 12 drops | *Cedar Virginia Red* |
| 42 drops | *BLEND* |

Make up your *BLEND* using the quantities above – store in a small dark glass bottle fitted with a dropper.

## AILMENT

Acne is caused by abnormal activity of the sebaceous glands which results in over production of sebum. This blocks the hair pores with a greasy plug. These sometimes show up as blackheads. Sebaceous glands appear to be affected by hormonal changes and stress, which can also trigger hormonal changes in the body. This is why acne is extremely common during puberty.

It is vital not to squeeze or damage the skin around affected areas as this can cause bacterial infection to become worse. This is when scarring occurs.

The *BLEND* treatments will help combat the bacterial infection and encourage the skin to heal.

The diet suggestions are aimed at encouraging the body to achieve a hormonal balance to stop the sebaceous glands over producing sebum.

It will take several months for the condition to improve so patience and perseverance is needed.

Do not use sunbeds and although sunlight will help do not over expose the skin as this can make the condition worse.

## SKIN APPLICATIONS

Make up a bottle of Acne Treatment Oil by adding 12 drops of *BLEND* to 30 ml of Jojoba Oil and 5 ml of Calendula Oil.

Also make up a bottle of Acne Treatment Lotion by adding 12 drops of *BLEND* to 30 ml of lotion.

Every night, sparingly apply the Acne Treatment Oil to the affected areas. Each morning sparingly apply the Acne Treatment Lotion to the affected areas.

For treatment during the day prepare cotton wool pads in the following way. Add 5 drops of *BLEND* to half a cup of spring water. Soak cotton wool pads in the water then squeeze them out and put into a small plastic bag. Gently wipe the affected skin with these pads every two hours.

Following these instructions will keep the skin protected from infection for the full 24 hours.

## BATHS

Add 8 drops of *BLEND* to your baths.

## DIET

Eat plenty of vegetables but only a modest amount of fruit. Avoid fatty foods, dairy foods and red meat as much as possible. Drink 7 glasses of water a day.

### Daily Supplements

| | |
|---|---|
| Vitamin A | dose as stated on container |
| Vitamin C | 1000 mgs |
| Zinc 30-40 | mgs |
| Vitamin E | 600 mgs |

# Anxiety

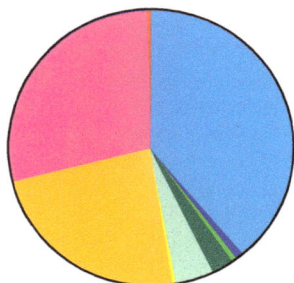

| | |
|---|---|
| esters | 39.0% |
| aliphatic aldehydes | 0.6% |
| ketones | trace |
| sesquiterpenes | 0.4% |
| lactones & coumarins | 2.6% |
| remainder | 4.9% |
| oxides | 0.1% |
| acids | trace |
| aromatic aldehydes | |
| monoterpenes | 23.2% |
| alcohols | 29.0% |
| phenols, phe. ethers | 0.2% |

**CCP of BLEND RECIPE**

*Bergamot* (citrus bergamia)

*Orange Petitgrain* (citrus aurantium amara)

*Rose Otto* (rosa damascena)

*Bergamot* is antispasmodic and calming. It is excellent for agitation and panic attacks. It is often the first choice in cases of depression. The aroma is light and citrus.

*Orange Petitgrain* is antispasmodic, calming and cheering. It is recommended in cases of nervous exhaustion. It also stimulates the immune system. The aroma is woody and floral.

*Rose Otto* calms anxiety. It has a sweet heavenly flowery aroma that lingers in the room. It relieves tension and feelings of inadequancy.

This blend of essential oils is particularly useful in relieving anxiety and tension. The strong aroma from *Rose Otto* is due to the damascenone.

*Chemical constituents to be found in the blend may include:*

- linalyl acetate, geranyl acetate, neryl acetate
- citral
- damascenone
- rose oxide

- $\alpha$-pinene, $\beta$-pinene, $\gamma$-terpinene, $\alpha$-terpinene, myrcene, limonene, stearoptene
- linalool, geraniol, $\alpha$-terpineol, nerol, citronellol, phenylethyl alcohol

## BLEND

| 21 drops | *Bergamot* |
|---|---|
| 14 drops | *Orange Petitgrain* |
| 7 drops | *Rose Otto* |
| 42 drops | *BLEND* |

Make up your *BLEND* using the quantities above – store in a small dark glass bottle fitted with a dropper.

## AILMENT

Continued anxiety upsets the balance between the various body functions. Conditions such as stomach ulcers and heart disease can be the result of unrelieved anxiety. A common physical symptom of anxiety is excess muscle tension. Massage treatment with the *BLEND* eases muscle tension and helps to calm anxious feelings.

It is important to identify and tackle the cause of the anxiety.

## MASSAGE

Make up a bottle of Anxiety Treatment Oil by adding 12 drops of *BLEND* to 30 ml of Sweet Almond Oil.

Take time to rest quietly and gently massage the treatment oil around your shoulders and neck. Even better lie face down on a couch and ask a friend or partner to gently massage your back. Another very good way to get relaxed is to simply have your feet gently rubbed or massaged with the Treatment Oil.

For real help in a case of chronic anxiety seek the professional help of an aromatherapist or reflexologist.

## BATHS

Add 8 drops of *BLEND* to your baths.

## VAPOURISERS

Add 5 drops of *BLEND* or 5 drops of Bergamot to a vapouriser. This is particularly helpful at night or on any occasion when anxiety threatens to cause a panic attack.

## TISSUE

Sprinkle 5 drops of *BLEND* onto a tissue. Wrap this up and keep in a pocket. Use it to inhale deeply whenever necessary.

## LIFE STYLE

Lack of fresh air, exercise and poor working conditions can lead to mental fatigue. Try to find time for outdoor activities. A daily walk can be really helpful. Relaxation, meditation and yoga are recommended. Also try to find a 'laugh' a day.

## DIET

Follow a balanced diet with plenty of fruit and vegetables. Avoid tea and coffee and any drinks with tannin in them.

### Daily Supplements
Vitamin B Complex as directed on the container
Vitamin C     250-500 mgs

# Athlete's Foot

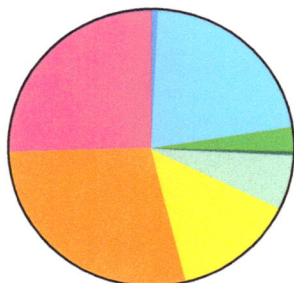

| | | |
|---|---|---|
| ■ | esters | 0.7% |
| ■ | aliphatic aldehydes | |
| ■ | ketones | 21.7% |
| ■ | sesquiterpenes | 3.0% |
| ■ | lactones & coumarins | 0.1% |
| ■ | remainder | 6.6% |
| ■ | oxides | 13.6% |
| ■ | acids | trace |
| ■ | aromatic aldehydes | |
| ■ | monoterpenes | 28.6% |
| ■ | alcohols | 25.7% |
| ■ | phenols, phe. ethers | |

## CCP of BLEND RECIPE

*Lavender Spike* (lavandula lactifolia)

*Tea Tree* (melaleuca alternifolia)

*Tagetes* (tagetes glandulifera)

*Lavender Spike* is antifungal and in general helpful with skin problems such as athlete's foot and ringworm.

*Tea Tree* is strongly antiseptic which helps to protect any skin wounds from infection. Recommended for boils, bites, cold sores, sweaty feet, athlete's foot and mouth ulcers.

*Tagetes* as well as helping athlete's foot to clear it is also useful for bunions, callouses and tired feet in general.

The ketones and alcohols will offer antifungal properties to this blend. The blend of the three oils attacks the condition and keeps the area free of infection.

*Chemical constituents to be found in the blend may include:*

- ■ linalyl acetate
- ■ tagetone, tagetenones, camphor
- ■ 1.8-cineole

- ■ α-pinene, γ-terpinene, limonene, α-terpinene, ocimene, terpinolene, *p*-cymene
- ■ terpinen-4-ol, α-terpineol, linalool

## BLEND

| 15 drops | *Lavender Spike* |
| 15 drops | *Tea Tree* |
| <u>15 drops</u> | *Tagetes* |
| <u>45 drops</u> | *BLEND* |

Make up your *BLEND* using the quantities above – store in a small dark glass bottle fitted with a dropper.

## AILMENT

Athlete's foot is the common name for a type of ringworm that infects the feet. The skin between the toes especially between the outer toes becomes infected with a microscopic fungus. It gets its name from the fact that it is often picked up in changing rooms of schools and sports clubs. The infected skin becomes thickened and moist. Eventually the skin becomes itchy and dries leading to cracking and peeling.

## LIFE STYLE

Always dry your feet thoroughly especially between the toes. Change socks and tights frequently. In fact if possible only wear cotton or wool garments.

## POWDER

Add 3 drops of the *BLEND* to a cup of talc. Mix it well. An electric blender with a fitted lid is ideal for this job. Powder the feet every day and place a little powder in all your footware.

## FOOT BATHS

Add 6 drops of *BLEND* to a bowl of warm water and soak feet every day. Dry well afterwards, particularly between the toes.

## APPLICATION

Make up a bottle of Athlete's Foot Treatment Oil by adding 4 drops of *BLEND* to 30 ml of Grapeseed Oil. Massage the feet with the Treatment Oil every night before going to bed. Make up a pot of Athlete's Foot Treatment Cream by adding 4 drops of *BLEND* to 30 ml of body and hand cream. Keep this Treatment Cream in the cupboard and use as a preventative measure. Apply to feet after visiting any place where you are likely to pick up the infection. In particular after visiting swimming pools and changing rooms.

# Baby Colic

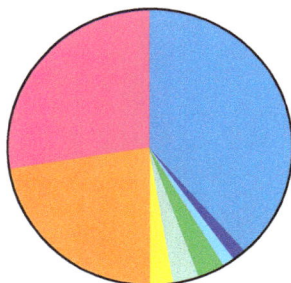

| | esters | 38.5% |
|---|---|---|
| | aliphatic aldehydes | 1.5% |
| | ketones | 1.5% |
| | sesquiterpenes | 3.0% |
| | lactones & coumarins | trace |
| | remainder | 3.0% |
| | oxides | 2.5% |
| | acids | trace |
| | aromatic aldehydes | |
| | monoterpenes | 22.5% |
| | alcohols | 27.5% |
| | phenols, phe. ethers | trace |

**CCP of BLEND RECIPE**

*Chamomile Roman* (chamaemelum nobile)

*Marjoram Sweet* (origanum majorana)

*Chamomile Roman* is a member of the compositae botanical family which is known to be generally soothing to the skin and calming to the digestive system. This oil is antispasmodic and calming. It is recommended for intestinal colic, flatulence and is helpful for jaundice and liver conditions. The aroma is fruity and apple like. This oil is an excellent oil for use with babies.

*Marjoram Sweet* has a spicy warm camphor like aroma. It is helpful in treating diarrhoea, enteritis and flatulence.

It can have powerful effects on hyperactivity being calming to the nervous system.

Known in folklore as 'joy of the mountain' it is associated with bringing peace and tranquillity.

*Chemical constituents to be found in the blend may include:*

- linalyl acetate, terpinyl acetate, geranyl acetate, angelates, tiglates, butyrates
- citral
- pinocarvone
- chamazulene, caryophyllene

- 1.8-cineole
- β-pinene, γ-terpinene, α-terpinene, limonene, myrcene, ocimene, p-cymene, sabinene
- farnesol, α-terpineol, linalool, terpinen-4-ol

## BLEND

10 drops  *Chamomile Roman*
10 drops  *Marjoram Sweet*
20 drops  *BLEND*

Make up your *BLEND* using the quantities above – store in a small dark glass bottle fitted with a dropper.

## AILMENT

Baby Colic is bouts of stomach pain that commonly affect young babies. It is very worrying to new mothers as the baby is often inconsolable until the griping pain ceases. The pain comes in waves over several hours and can recur regularly each day. A variety of factors are thought to be the cause of this distress which normally eases up as the baby grows. If attacks are prolonged consult a doctor for advice.

## TREATMENT

Make sure the baby's feeding times are relaxed and peaceful. Try to prevent the baby from feeding too quickly as they may take in air with the milk causing flatulence. Make sure that the baby is well 'winded' during and after the feed.

The more peaceful and regular the baby's routine is the greater chance that the colic attacks will gradually subside.

Keep the baby's room at a steady temperature so that the baby neither overheats nor becomes chilly.

## APPLICATION

Make up a bottle of Baby Colic Treatment Oil by adding 2 drops of *BLEND* to 30 ml of Sunflower Oil.

If the baby has colic after feeding rub this Treatment Oil sparingly around your baby's tummy. Use very gentle clockwise stroking. This will help to calm the baby. Turn the baby over and repeat the gentle circular movements over the middle of the baby's back.

## VAPOURISER

Place a bowl of steaming water in the baby's room, well away from the baby's head. Add 1 drop of *BLEND* to the water. This allows the molecules of essential oils to evaporate and circulate through the room.

You can also use 1 drop of *Dill (anethum graveolens)* in the same manner. *Dill* is used in commercial gripe water.

## DIET

If you are breast feeding your baby your own diet is important. Avoid wine, citrus fruits, grapes and fried onions. These have been known to be the cause of the problem.

# Baby Coughs and Colds

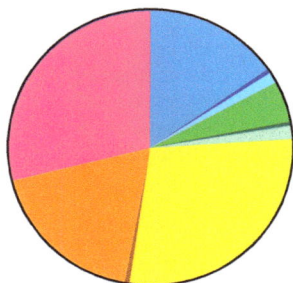

| | | |
|---|---|---|
| | esters | 15.3% |
| | aliphatic aldehydes | 0.3% |
| | ketones | 1.7% |
| | sesquiterpenes | 5.0% |
| | lactones & coumarins | 0.1% |
| | remainder | 1.6% |
| | oxides | 28.4% |
| | acids | trace |
| | aromatic aldehydes | 0.3% |
| | monoterpenes | 18.3% |
| | alcohols | 29.0% |
| | phenols, phe. ethers | trace |

**CCP of BLEND RECIPE**

*Lavender True* (lavandula angustifolia)

*Tea Tree* (melaleuca alternifolia)

*Eucalyptus Blue Gum* (eucalyptus globulus)

*Lavender True* is antiviral, bactericidal and antiseptic. It offers help to treating bronchitis, coughs, sinusitis and TB. Its beautiful familiar aroma is soothing and calming.

*Tea Tree* is strongly antiseptic and bactericidal – excellent for clearing up infections.

*Eucalyptus Blue Gum* is a decongestant, expectorant, mucolytic. It is used to treat asthma, catarhh, diphtheria, laryngitis, pneumonia, scarlet fever and tonsillitis.

A well balanced chemical blend. Four families take the major share of the oil. The oxides offer help with the congestion of mucous. The esters help to calm the system and the alcohols and monoterpenes can act as tonics.

*Chemical constituents to be found in the blend may include:*

- linalyl acetate, lavandulyl acetate
- citral
- pinocarvone
- β-caryophyllene, viridiflorene, aromadendrene
- coumarin
- 1.8-cineole
- α-pinene, α-terpinene, γ-terpinene, *p*-cymene, terpinolene
- α-terpineol, terpinen-4-ol, borneol, globulol, lavandulol

## BLEND

| 6 drops | *Lavender True* |
|---------|----------------|
| 6 drops | *Tea Tree* |
| 6 drops | *Eucalyptus Blue Gum* |
| 18 drops | *BLEND* |

Make up your *BLEND* using the quantities above – store in a small dark glass bottle fitted with a dropper.

## TREATMENT

Continuous coughs and cold are distressing both to mother and baby. Some precautions can help to alleviate the frequency of these conditions.

Put 2 drops of *BLEND* into a plant spray full of water. Use this to regularly spray rooms in the home – this will fend off infections. Do not use this spray directly in the baby's room. To help your baby cope with the congestion of the nasal passages place a bowl of warm water under the baby's cot (away from the head end) and add 1 drop of *BLEND* to the water. The vapour carries the molecules around the room and this gently eases the baby's congestion.

## TISSUES

If the baby is very stuffed up take a tissue and put 1 drop of *BLEND* on it. Place the tissue safely under the top sheet of the cot.

## BATHS

Add 1 drop of *BLEND* to baby's bath water. Swish it round well.

## MASSAGE

Make up a bottle of Baby Coughs and Colds Treatment Oil by adding 1 drop of *BLEND* to 15 ml of Sunflower Oil.

Massage the baby's chest and back with gentle circular movements.

It is a good idea to do this just before bedtime.

Do not continue the treatments for more than a week at a time.

## LIFE STYLE

Provided the baby is well wrapped and protected from cold weather a regular outing in the fresh air will help with the congestion and discomfort that comes with a cold.

# Baby Fretful

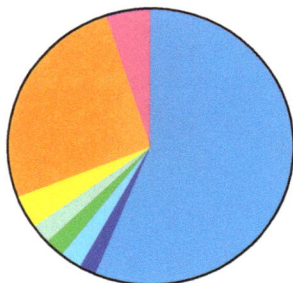

| | | |
|---|---|---|
| | esters | 56.5% |
| | aliphatic aldehydes | 1.8% |
| | ketones | 2.3% |
| | sesquiterpenes | 2.3% |
| | lactones & coumarins | trace |
| | remainder | 2.3% |
| | oxides | 3.7% |
| | acids | trace |
| | aromatic aldehydes | |
| | monoterpenes | 26.2% |
| | alcohols | 4.9% |
| | phenols, phe. ethers | trace |

**CCP of BLEND RECIPE**

 *Chamomile Roman* (chamaemelum nobile)

 *Mandarin* (citrus reticulata)

*Chamomile Roman* is a calming sedative oil. It helps with insomnia and irritability. It is highly respected for its calming influence on all systems. It has a fruity apple like aroma. This is a very safe oil most suitable to use with babies and children.

*Mandarin* is especially good for use with children. It has revitalising properties and helps combat insomnia and anxiety. The fruit was given to the Mandarins as a sign of respect – hence its name. The oil has a sweet sharp floral aroma. It is a member of the rutaceae botanical family which is known to generally aid digestion and skin conditions.

The large proportion of esters in this blend indicates a calming effect will be experienced. Its monoterpenes may well ease digestive problems. The two oils blend well together.

*Chemical constituents to be found in the blend may include:*

- angelates, tiglates, butyrates, methyl anthranilate
- citral
- pinocarvone
- caryophyllene, chamazulene
- 1.8-cineole
- α-pinene, γ-terpinene, limonene, myrcene, *p*-cymene
- α-terpineol, farnesol, linalool, citronellol

## BLEND

| 30 drops | *Chamomile Roman* |
|----------|-------------------|
| 10 drops | *Mandarin* |
| 40 drops | *BLEND* |

Make up your *BLEND* using the quantities above – store in a small dark glass bottle fitted with a dropper.

## AILMENT

Fretfulness as a frequent occurrence is very upsetting for everyone. With very young babies it is difficult to decide when the baby has wind, colic, teething pain or a condition that needs medical attention.

If the baby is not hungry or wet check for any other obvious reasons for the baby's discontent. Often loud background noises such as TV or a wrong ambient temperature cause frustration.

Fretful periods tend to decrease if the baby's routine is as peaceful and regular as possible.

## FEET

Touch is a wonderful way to ease any anxiety state but you want to avoid continuous cuddling being the only way to comfort your baby. An alternative way is to gently massage the baby's feet. This may sound strange but it is a method handed down from ancient cultures and one adopted by many trained nannies. Make up a bottle of Baby Fretful Treatment Oil by adding 4 drops of *BLEND* to 30 ml of Sunflower Oil.

Lay the baby down and rub a little of the Treatment Oil on the baby's feet. Grasp each foot firmly between your thumbs and fingers. Gently massage both feet, simultaneously, by moving your thumbs in a circular rhythmic motion from the centre of the foot to the base of the toes. The baby may well fidget to start with but will usually settle quite quickly and often be comforted to sleep.

You can also use this action to just comfort a baby over his socks or garment without the Treatment Oil.

## VAPOURISER

If the baby is fretful at night place a bowl of warm water under the cot but not directly beneath the baby's head. Place 1 drop of *BLEND* in the water. The oil molecules will circulate and have a calming effect.

## MASSAGE

A baby enjoys a massage as part of his contact with his parents. Lay the baby in a warm and comfortable position. Using the Treatment Oil gently massage the baby with soft circular strokes. In other words caress your baby and softly sing or talk to them. Spend a little time with the baby lying on his tummy and then a little time on his back. Gently stroke his little limbs.

# Baby Nappy Rash

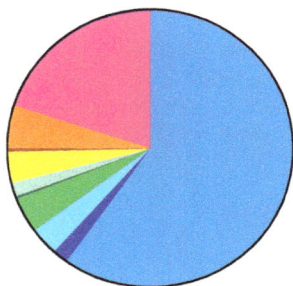

| | | |
|---|---|---|
| | esters | 60.0% |
| | aliphatic aldehydes | 1.5% |
| | ketones | 3.5% |
| | sesquiterpenes | 4.0% |
| | lactones & coumarins | 0.1% |
| | remainder | 1.9% |
| | oxides | 3.5% |
| | acids | trace |
| | aromatic aldehydes | 0.5% |
| | monoterpenes | 4.5% |
| | alcohols | 20.5% |
| | phenols, phe. ethers | trace |

**CCP of BLEND RECIPE**

*Lavender True* (lavandula angustifolia)

*Chamomile Roman* (chamaemelum nobile)

*Lavender True* is excellent for the regeneration of skin cells. It heals wounds and scars and is on the whole a calming oil. It is antifungal and bactericidal. It can help with burns, eczema, herpes, psoriasis, spots and wounds.

*Chamomile Roman* is a member of the compositae botanical family which is known to be generally soothing to the skin and calming to the digestive system. This oil can be used to treat cracked nipples, psoriasis, skin irritations and. surgical scars.

These two oils are particularly suitable for use with young babies. This blend with its large proportion of esters is soothing and calming both to the spirit and to the skin.

*Chemical constituents to be found in the blend may include:*

- linalyl acetate, lavandulyl acetate, angelates, tiglates, butyrates
- citral
- pinocarvone, camphor
- chamazulene, β-caryophyllene
- coumarin
- 1.8-cineole
- cuminaldehyde, benzyl aldehyde
- α-pinene, sabinene
- terpinen-4-ol, α-terpineol, linalool, farnesol, lavandulol

## BLEND

| | |
|---|---|
| 8 drops | *Lavender True* |
| 8 drops | *Chamomile Roman* |
| 16 drops | *BLEND* |

Make up your *BLEND* using the quantities above – store in a small dark glass bottle fitted with a dropper.

## AILMENT

Most babies suffer from nappy/diaper rash at some time. It is an angry red rash caused by the baby's urine. It is painful and worrying to the baby and needs immediate treatment. Make sure that nappies are never left wet for long. Untreated nappy rash can give rise to fungal infection which causes the skin to become raw and painful. Essential oils are excellent in dealing with this problem.

## APPLICATION

Before changing the baby's nappy prepare a bowl of warm water. For each pint of water in the bowl add 1 drop of *BLEND*. Use clean cotton wool pads to gently sponge the baby's bottom.

Make up a pot of Baby Nappy Rash Treatment Ointment by adding 4 drops of *BLEND* to 40 ml of Zinc and Castor Oil ointment (see Home Pharmacy).

After washing the baby's bottom make sure it is thoroughly dry and apply the treatment ointment carefully making sure that all areas affected by the rash have been covered.

## LIFE STYLE

Change nappies frequently and always give the baby a short time without a nappy on. Air is a natural healer and the baby will enjoy the freedom.

If the nappy rash is severe the skin looks as though it has been burned or scalded. In this case avoid using any plastic protection and use washable pure cotton nappies until the skin heals. When washing the nappies place 6 drops of *BLEND* in the softener used in the rinse cycle of your washing machine or add 2 drops of *BLEND* to rinse water if washing the nappies by hand.

## BATHS

Add 1 drop of *BLEND* to the baby's bath.

## OTHER OILS

Other oils that are helpful to damaged skin are *Sandalwood* (santalum album) and *Eucalyptus Lemon Scented* (eucalyptus citriodora)

You can substitute these oils for the ones used in the *BLEND* if you wish.

107

# Baby Teething

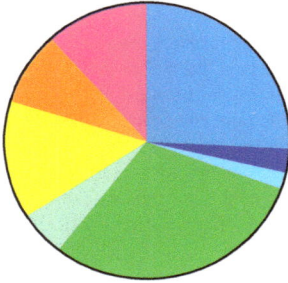

| | | |
|---|---|---|
| | esters | 25.7% |
| | aliphatic aldehydes | 2.3% |
| | ketones | 1.7% |
| | sesquiterpenes | 31.0% |
| | lactones & coumarins | trace |
| | remainder | 5.2% |
| | oxides | 13.8% |
| | acids | trace |
| | aromatic aldehydes | |
| | monoterpenes | 8.7% |
| | alcohols | 11.6% |
| | phenols, phe. ethers | trace |

## CCP of BLEND RECIPE

*Chamomile Roman* (chamaemelum nobile)

*Chamomile German* (matricaria recutica)

*Ginger* (zingiber officinale)

*Chamomile Roman* is an antiinflammatory, eases pain and is calming to the whole system. It soothes irritability and acts as a general sedative.

*Chamomile German* is an analgesic bringing relief for the pain. It is recommended in particular for toothache and skin rashes. It also calms the digestive system.

*Ginger* is an analgesic and temperature reducing. It is good for toothache catarrh, chronic bronchitis and for all side effects of colds. It has a warm pleasant spicy aroma and is to be found in many ancient recipes.

This blend with its large proportion of the ester and sesquiterpene families present offers a calming effect. The oils combine well to treat the pain, lower the temperature and fight any infection.

*Chemical constituents to be found in the blend may include:*

- angelates, tiglates, butyrates
- geranial
- pinocarvone, gingerone
- chamazulene, farnesene, caryophyllene, β-sesquiphellandrene zingiberene, *ar*-curcumene

- α-bisabolol oxide, 1.8-cineole
- α-pinene, β-pinene, camphene
- α-bisabolol, α-terpineol, linalool, citronellol, gingerol

**BLEND**

| 5 drops | *Chamomile Roman* |
|---|---|
| 5 drops | *Chamomile German* |
| 5 drops | *Ginger* |
| 15 drops | *BLEND* |

Make up your *BLEND* using the quantities above – store in a small dark glass bottle fitted with a dropper.

**AILMENT**

By the time a child reaches 2 to 3 years they will have cut their 20 milk teeth. Children vary greatly as to when the teeth arrive. Some babies do not get any teeth until after their first birthday whereas very occasionally a baby is actually born with teeth. The normal pattern is for the first tooth to appear at about 6 months old.

Some babies suffer quite severe symptoms of raised temperature, runny noses and runny stools with a show of considerable discomfort. Other babies seem hardly to notice and their teeth appear with no problems at all.

Disturbed nights result in tiredness and irritation and can set up a vicious circle of upset that is difficult to break. The following treatments will help to break this cycle.

**TREATMENT**

Make up a bottle of Baby Teething Treatment Oil by adding 2 drops of *BLEND* to 30 ml of Sweet Almond Oil.

Collect a little of the Treatment Oil onto your fingers and thumb and gently massage the baby's cheek running down the jaw line in soft comforting strokes.

To help ease the soreness of the baby's gums place 1 teaspoonful of the Treatment Oil into a small cup of ice cold water. Take a cotton bud and dip it into the prepared water. Gently wipe the baby's gums with the cotton bud.

Alternatively you can put just one drop of *Chamomile Roman* into a large cup of ice cold water. Swish the water around thoroughly so that the oil mixes well. Now apply to the baby's gum with a cotton bud in the same way as above.

Do not put more than 1 drop of *Roman Chamomile* in the water – if more than 1 drop falls in by accident throw the water away and start again.

**FEET**

To help the baby settle you can use the foot massage recommended for fretful behaviour.

Grasp each foot firmly between your thumbs and fingers. Gently massage both feet, simultaneously, by moving your thumbs in a circular rhythmic motion from the centre of the foot to the base of the toes. The baby may well fidget to start with but will usually settle quite quickly and often be comforted to sleep. You can do this over the baby's socks or baby suit at any time the baby is restless.

# Back Pain

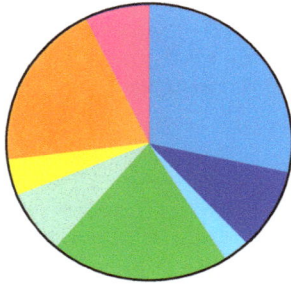

| | | |
|---|---|---|
| ■ | esters | 28.5% |
| ■ | aliphatic aldehydes | 9.4% |
| ■ | ketones | 3.5% |
| ■ | sesquiterpenes | 20.2% |
| ■ | lactones & coumarins | trace |
| ■ | remainder | 7.6% |
| ■ | oxides | 3.9% |
| ■ | acids | trace |
| ■ | aromatic aldehydes | |
| ■ | monoterpenes | 19.8% |
| ■ | alcohols | 7.1% |
| ■ | phenols, phe. ethers | |

**CCP of BLEND RECIPE**

 *Chamomile Roman* (chamaemelum nobile)

 *Eucalyptus Staigeriana* (eucalyptus staigeriana)

 *Ginger* (zingiber officinale)

*Chamomile Roman* is potent sedative as well as being a long lasting antiiflammatory. It is highly respected for its calming influence on all systems. It relieves muscular pain and is recommended for back pain, gout and also period pains.

*Eucalyptus Staigeriana* is a gentle member of the eucalyptus family. It has a light lemon aroma in contrast to the harsher camphor aroma of many eucalyptus oils. It is an antiinflammatory recommended for back pain, neck ache and muscle cramps.

*Ginger* with its warm spicy aroma is recommended for arthritis, back spasms, rheumatism and all side effects of colds.

These oils give a well-balanced blend of the chemical families.

---

*Chemical constituents to be found in the blend may include:*

■ angelates, tiglates, butyrates, menthyl acetate

■ neral, geranial, citronellal

■ pinocarvone, gingerone

■ 1.8-cineole

■ chamazulene, caryophyllene, zingibe-rene, β-sesquiphellandrene, *ar*-curcu-mene

■ α-pinene, limonene

■ α-terpineol, nerol, citronellol, borneol, linalool, gingerol

## BLEND

| | |
|---|---|
| 14 drops | *Chamomile Roman* |
| 14 drops | *Eucalyptus Staigeriana* |
| 14 drops | *Ginger* |
| 42 drops | *BLEND* |

Make up your *BLEND* using the quantities above – store in a small dark glass bottle fitted with a dropper.

## AILMENT

Backache is one of the common chronic conditions that Doctors are asked to deal with. Its possible causes are numerous. Many causes are not serious but occasionally backache can indicate serious problems which need to be identified. The most likely cause is mechanical strain on the back itself. Often the exact reason for the pain is difficult to pin down. Faulty posture or an awkward movement may have stretched ligaments. One common cause of back strain is leaning over at right angles and lifting a heavy weight. Extreme pain may indicate that there is a slipped disc or cracked vertebrae. These severe injuries take several months to heal.

## MASSAGE

Back massage with essential oils can be very beneficial to sufferers of chronic back pain. The oils penetrate deeply into muscle tissue and assist the body's natural healing processes. The combination of the oils and gentle body massage bring a good flow of blood to the damaged tissues.

Make up a bottle of Back Pain Treatment Oil by adding 12 drops of *BLEND* to 30 ml of Sweet Almond Oil. Lie flat on the couch and get a friend to gently massage your back with long flowing strokes with the Treatment Oil. For self treatment you can massage your lower back and around your neck and shoulders. This will

still benefit you as the oils are being absorbed into your blood stream.

For chronic sufferers of back pain it is strongly recommended that you book regular appointments with an aromatherapist.

## BATHS

Add 8 drops of *BLEND* to your baths.

## COMPRESSES

Use hot and cold compresses to alleviate severe pain. Prepare two bowls of water one as warm as you can bear and the other ice cold. Place 4 drops of *BLEND* in each bowl. Soak your compress cloths in each of the bowls. Wring out each cloth and apply alternatively to the painful area. This will increase the flow of blood to the area.

## LIFE STYLE

As the major cause of back ache is poor posture, Alexander Technique sessions have an excellent record in helping sufferers. It is highly recommended – try to attend for treatment at least once a week to start with.

# Blood Pressure High

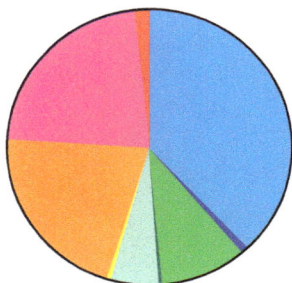

| | |
|---|---|
| esters | 38.1% |
| aliphatic aldehydes | 0.7% |
| ketones | trace |
| sesquiterpenes | 9.6% |
| lactones & coumarins | 0.3% |
| remainder | 5.0% |
| oxides | 0.4% |
| acids | trace |
| aromatic aldehydes | |
| monoterpenes | 22.2% |
| alcohols | 22.0% |
| phenols, phe. ethers | 1.7% |

**CCP of BLEND RECIPE**

*Clary Sage* (salvia sclarea)

*Lemon* (citrus limon)

*Marjoram Sweet* (origanum majorana)

*Ylang Ylang* (cananga odorata)

*Clary Sage* is recommended for high blood pressure and high cholesterol, phlebitis and varicose veins. It is a soothing, calming oil. It has a nutty earthy aroma.

*Lemon* is a diuretic and helps with obesity, lowers blood pressure and stems bleeding. It is a general rejuvenator due to its oxidising agents.

*Marjoram Sweet* is a diuretic, vasodilator and balances heart and circulation. It is calming to the nervous system.

*Ylang Ylang* helps with panic and shock. It slows the heart beat and breathing rate. It has a sweet heavy exotic aroma.

*Chemical constituents to be found in the blend may include:*

- linalyl acetate, geranyl acetate, terpinyl acetate, benzyl acetate
- citral
- caryophyllene, germacrene
- bergaptene
- α-pinene, β-pinene, γ-terpinene, α-terpinene, limonene, myrcene, p-cymene, sabinene, ocimene
- sclareol, linalool, terpinen-4-ol, α-terpineol
- methyl eugenol

## BLEND

| | |
|---|---|
| 21 drops | *Clary Sage* |
| 7 drops | *Lemon* |
| 7 drops | *Marjoram Sweet* |
| 7 drops | *Ylang Ylang* |
| 42 drops | *BLEND* |

Make up your *BLEND* using the quantities above – store in a small dark glass bottle fitted with a dropper.

## BLOOD PRESSURE

Blood pressure is expressed as the systolic / diastolic readings.

A typical reading is 120 / 70. Normal blood pressure is considered to lie between the following range:

(100 to 140) / (60 to 90).

## AILMENT

Most cases of high blood pressure have no recognised cause and are known as primary hypertension. Blood pressure that is persistently higher than would be expected should be taken as a warning as it can affect the adequate functioning of the body's organs, for example the kidneys. Some factors, that can be controlled, are often the cause of high blood pressure. For instance – obesity, heavy drinking and smoking. Raised blood pressure definitely shortens life span so it is important to review and correct all possible causes.

## BATHS

Add 8 drops of *BLEND* to your baths.

## MASSAGE

Make up a bottle of High Blood Pressure Treatment Oil by adding 12 drops of *BLEND* to 30 ml of Sweet Almond Oil.

Get a friend to massage your back with this Treatment Oil. Lie on a couch in a warm room. The massage should be slow, gentle circular movements from the base of the back to the top. A regular visit to an aromatherapist is recommended as it is extremely important to return your blood pressure to its normal level.

## LIFE STYLE

Take complete stock of your life style. Cut out smoking and fatty foods. Drink no more than one glass of red wine a day. Attend regular relaxation classes and remove as much stress from your life as possible. Consult the treatments recommended for Anxiety. Make sure that you have time for leisure and relaxation and that you take regular gentle exercise. Also rest with your feet raised whenever possible.

## DIET

Reduce your intake of salt. Follow a low fat diet to ensure that your cholesterol level is kept low.

**Supplements**
Multi vitamin/mineral tablet B Complex as per container
Vitamin C 1000 mgs twice a day
Garlic capsules as per container
Evening Primrose Oil – 2 tablets daily

# Blood Pressure Low

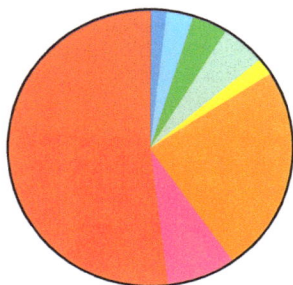

| | | |
|---|---|---|
| ■ | esters | 1.8% |
| ■ | aliphatic aldehydes | trace |
| ■ | ketones | 3.6% |
| ■ | sesquiterpenes | 4.0% |
| ■ | lactones & coumarins | |
| ■ | remainder | 4.8% |
| ■ | oxides | 2.0% |
| ■ | acids | trace |
| ■ | aromatic aldehydes | trace |
| ■ | monoterpenes | 24.0% |
| ■ | alcohols | 7.8% |
| ■ | phenols, phe. ethers | 52.0% |

**CCP of BLEND RECIPE**

*Clove Bud* (syzygium aromaticum)

*Pine Scotch* (pinus sylvestris)

*Thyme Red* (thymus vulgaris thymoliferum)

*Clove Bud* is analgesic, antiviral, bactericidal and stimulating. It is used in many modern pharmaceuticals. Used in traditional medicine for alleviating toothache. It raises blood pressure and regulates the thyroid gland. The oil has a strong spicy aroma.

*Pine Scotch* is bactericidal, a decongestant and raises blood pressure. It is credited with hormone like behaviour similar to cortisone. It has a fresh forest aroma.

*Thyme Red* is a strongly stimulating oil. It stimulates the capillaries and raises blood pressure and helps with anaemia. It is a general and neurotonic offering help with depression and stress.

This oil should be avoided during pregnancy.

---

*Chemical constituents to be found in the blend may include:*

- ■ bornyl acetate, terpinyl acetate
- ■ cryptone, camphor, thujone
- ■ β-caryophyllene
- ■ humulene oxide, 1.8-cineole

- ■ α-pinene, β-pinene, γ-terpinene, limonene, myrcene, sabinene
- ■ terpinen-4-ol, linalool, borneol
- ■ eugenol, aceteugenol, thymol, carvacrol

## BLEND

16 drops   *Clove Bud*
 8 drops   *Pine Scotch*
16 drops   *Thyme Red*
40 drops   *BLEND*

Make up your *BLEND* using the quantities above – store in a small dark glass bottle fitted with a dropper.

## BLOOD PRESSURE

Blood pressure is expressed as the systolic / diastolic readings.

A typical reading is 120 / 70. Normal blood pressure is considered to lie between the following range:

(100 to 140) / (60 to 90).

## AILMENT

Low blood pressure (hypotension) is not considered as serious as high blood pressure (hypertension) and is rarely a chronic condition. Indeed in this country it is rarely given as a medical diagnosis. However in some countries it is widely identified and probably is used for cases of extreme lassitude with no obvious cause. Low blood pressure can occur after a severe shock causing giddiness and fainting. Another symptom is a feeling of giddiness on standing up quickly – more common amongst the elderly. Certain essential oils help to restore normal blood pressure as they can balance the blood circulation.

## BATHS

Add 8 drops of *BLEND* to your baths.

## MASSAGE

Make up a bottle of Low Blood Pressure Treatment Oil by adding 12 drops of *BLEND* to 30 ml of Sweet Almond Oil.

Massage your lower back and the soles of your feet. The Treatment Oil will stimulate the body's immune system and strengthen its resistance. Low blood pressure can occur if the adrenal glands are functioning below par – *Pine Scotch* is recommended for balancing the action of the adrenal glands. *Clove Bud* balances the action of the thyroid gland and *Thyme Red* helps with circulation and stimulates the white corpuscles. This Treatment Oil can also be used to help with ME (Myalgic Encephalomylitis).

## LIFE STYLE

Take plenty of regular rest and gentle exercise. Build up your strength gradually, do not rush into extra activities until you are able to cope happily with them.

## DIET

Follow a diet of whole foods. Avoid tea, coffee, alcohol and tobacco.

### Supplements

Vitamin E     200 I.U.s daily
Vitamin C     1000 mgs daily
Iron tablets as per container

# Breast Abscess

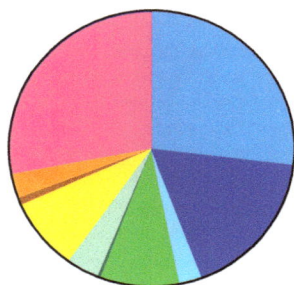

| | | |
|---|---|---|
| | esters | 27.6% |
| | aliphatic aldehydes | 16.6% |
| | ketones | 2.4% |
| | sesquiterpenes | 10.0% |
| | lactones & coumarins | 0.2% |
| | remainder | 3.6% |
| | oxides | 8.4% |
| | acids | |
| | aromatic aldehydes | 0.6% |
| | monoterpenes | 2.6% |
| | alcohols | 28.0% |
| | phenols, phe. ethers | trace |

**CCP of BLEND RECIPE**

 *Lavender True* (lavandula angustifolia)

 *Chamomile German* (matricaria recutica)

 *Eucalyptus Lemon Scented* (eucalyptus citriodora)

*Lavender True* is excellent for the regeneration of skin cells. It heals wounds and scars and is on the whole a calming oil.

*Chamomile German* is bactericidal and a decongestant. It helps to lower temperature and assists the skin to heal. It is recommended for various skin disturbances such as psoriasis, rashes, burns, boils, spots and so on.

*Eucalyptus Lemon Scented* has a fragrant lemon tinged aroma. It has a general calming effect and helps to abate a feverish state. It is used to treat many types of skin damage for example chicken-pox sores, wounds and herpes.

*Chemical constituents to be found in the blend may include:*

- linalyl acetate, lavandulyl acetate, citronellyl acetate
- citronellal
- camphor
- caryophyllene, chamazulene
- coumarin

- 1.8-cineole, α-bisabolol oxide
- cuminaldehyde, benzaldehyde
- α-pinene
- citronellol, α-bisabolol, borneol, α-terpineol, terpinen-4-ol, lavandulol

## BLEND

| 15 drops | *Lavender True* |
|---|---|
| 5 drops | *Chamomile German* |
| 5 drops | *Eucalyptus Lemon Scented* |
| 25 drops | *BLEND* |

Make up your *BLEND* using the quantities above – store in a small dark glass bottle fitted with a dropper.

## AILMENT

Mastitis is inflammation of the breast generally due to nipples becoming sore and damaged. If it does not clear up quickly an abscess can form. An abscess is a collection of pus due to the action of bacterial infection. Essential oils are excellent for helping to fight bacterial infections. If an breast abscess forms during lactation it will be necessary to stop feeding the baby from the infected breast until the infection is cleared. To relieve the pressure, removal of milk from the infected breast can be done gently by hand.

## TREATMENT

Apply just 2 drops of neat *Lavender True* to the abscess itself. Next prepare a bowl of warm water and add 5 drops of *BLEND* to it. Make a compress by soaking a clean cotton cloth in the prepared water. Wring the cloth out and wrap gently around the breast. The warmth is comforting. Keep the water warm and repeat this when the breast is giving discomfort. Make up a bottle of Breast Abscess Treatment Oil by adding 12 drops of *BLEND* to 30 ml of Sweet Almond Oil. Apply this Treatment Oil to both breasts, gently massaging them. If you are still feeding from the uninfected breast be sure to wash the nipple thoroughly to remove all the essential oil before feeding the baby. If the abscess does not heal and you have a high temperature consult your doctor. He may decide to prescribe antibiotics – this will mean that breast feeding will have to stop for a while. It can be difficult to re-establish it.

## LIFE STYLE

To prevent cracked and damaged nipples occurring take advice from your midwife who will assist you to encourage the baby to fasten correctly on the nipple.

After each feed apply the Treatment Oil gently to both breasts and nipples. Always wash the nipples well before feeding the baby.

Geranium leaves can be very soothing and healing if you start to develop sore nipples. Wrap the geranium leaf, furry side to the skin, around your nipple. You can just tuck them inside your bra. They will tingle a little. If, however, you find that they actually irritate the skin stop using them.

# Bronchitis

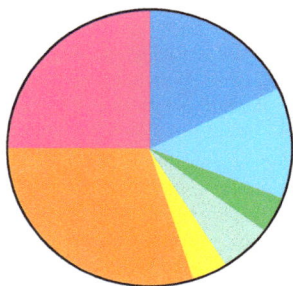

| | | |
|---|---|---|
| ■ | esters | 18.7% |
| ■ | aliphatic aldehydes | 0.5% |
| ■ | ketones | 12.0% |
| ■ | sesquiterpenes | 3.8% |
| ■ | lactones & coumarins | trace |
| ■ | remainder | 6.2% |
| ■ | oxides | 4.8% |
| ■ | acids | trace |
| ■ | aromatic aldehydes | |
| ■ | monoterpenes | 29.2% |
| ■ | alcohols | 24.8% |
| ■ | phenols, phe. ethers | |

## CCP of BLEND RECIPE

 *Eucalyptus Dives* (eucalyptus dives)

 *Tea Tree* (melaleuca alternifolia)

 *Chamomile Roman* (chamaemelum nobile)

*Eucalyptus Dives* is an expectorant, decongestant and mucolytic. It is helpful in relieving bronchitis, catarrh and sinusitis. Avoid in pregnancy and with young children. You can substitute it with *eucalyptus staigeriana* for a gentler action.

*Tea Tree* is strongly bactericidal and is most effective at clearing infections. It is recommended for asthma, bronchitis, catarrh and whooping cough.

*Chamomile Roman* reduces temperatures and fevers, and generally relaxes the whole body. It is helpful for nervous asthma, irritability, neuralgia and migraines.

---

*Chemical constituents to be found in the blend may include:*

■ angelates, tiglates, butyrates
■ piperitone, pinocarvone
■ β-caryophyllene, chamazulene, aromadendrene, viridiflorene, cadinene
■ 1.8-cineole

■ α-pinene, *p*-cymene, limonene, α-phellandrene, γ-terpinene, α-terpinene, camphene, thujene
■ α-terpineol, terpinen-4-ol, linalool, globulol, piperitol, viridiflorol, farnesol, *trans*-pinocarveol, nerolidol

## BLEND

| | |
|---|---|
| 10 drops | *Eucalyptus Dives* |
| 20 drops | *Tea Tree* |
| 10 drops | *Chamomile Roman* |
| 40 drops | *BLEND* |

Make up your *BLEND* using the quantities above – store in a small dark glass bottle fitted with a dropper.

## AILMENT

Acute bronchitis is due to the spread of a viral infection from the nose and throat, commonly referred to as a cold settling on the chest. The bronchi are much more vulnerable to infection if they are irritated by smoke and fumes and in some cases even by cold air. A dry uncomfortable cough develops and a fever shows. The inflammation is caused by the over production of mucous in the bronchial tubes. The virus will run its course but essential oils can alleviate the discomfort.

Chronic bronchitis is a much more serious condition accounting for the death of 20,000 people a year in this country. The inflammation of the bronchi becomes very established and the lung tissue receives permanent damage. The efficiency of the lungs becomes impaired and they have difficulty in maintaining the correct levels of oxygen for the body. The major causes of chronic bronchitis are smoking and air pollution.

## BATHS

Add 8 drops of *BLEND* to your baths.

## TISSUES

Place 3 drops of *BLEND* onto a tissue and inhale deeply. Carry a few prepared tissues in your pocket to use when required.

## APPLICATION

Make up a bottle of Bronchitis Treatment Oil by adding 12 drops of *BLEND* to 30 ml of Sweet Almond Oil.

Rub the Treatment Oil over your chest and back first thing in the morning and last thing at night. The essential oils will enter your blood stream and circulate around the infected lung area helping to clear the congestion and fight the infection.

## LIFE STYLE

It is vital not to smoke and to keep away from polluted air. Do not stay in smoke polluted rooms.

## DIET

Good foods are vegetables and vegetable soups, pulses, whole grains and all salad foods except for tomatoes. Cut down on dairy foods as they encourage the production of mucous. Avoid bacon, pork and ham. Drink 8 glasses of spring water daily.

### Daily Supplements

Multi vitamin/mineral tablet
| | |
|---|---|
| Vitamin B6 | 50 mgs |
| Vitamin A | 5000 I.U.s |
| Vitamin C | 1000 mgs |

Six Kelp Tablets

# Bursitis

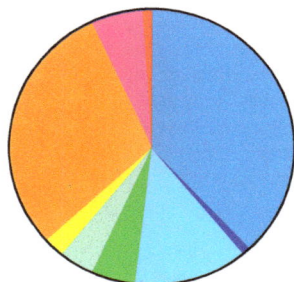

| | | |
|---|---|---|
| | esters | 38.0% |
| | aliphatic aldehydes | 1.0% |
| | ketones | 13.0% |
| | sesquiterpenes | 5.0% |
| | lactones & coumarins | trace |
| | remainder | 4.0% |
| | oxides | 2.7% |
| | acids | trace |
| | aromatic aldehydes | |
| | monoterpenes | 29.5% |
| | alcohols | 5.8% |
| | phenols, phe. ethers | 1.0% |

**CCP of BLEND RECIPE**

*Hyssop* (hyssopus officinalis)

*Juniper Berry* (juniperus communis)

*Chamomile Roman* (chamaemelum nobile)

*Hyssop* is antiinflammatory, antiseptic and a sedative. It helps bruises, dissolves boils and swellings and is recommended for rheumatism. This oil should be avoided in cases of epilepsy and also should not be used during pregnancy.

*Juniper Berry* is a diuretic and is particularly useful in clearing fluid retention. It is recommended for cellulite, obesity, oedema, painful joints, psoriasis and stiffness. This oil is a powerful detoxifying agent. It helps to eliminate uric acid from the system. Avoid during pregnancy and do not use if kidneys are inflamed.

*Chamomile Roman* is recommended for gout. It will also exert a soothing influence on the whole system.

*Chemical constituents to be found in the blend may include:*

- bornyl acetate, methyl myrtenate, angelates, tiglates, butyrates
- pinocamphone, isopinocamphone, pinocarvone, camphor
- caryophyllene, cadinene, humulenes, chamazulene, germacrene
- umbelliferone
- 1.8-cineole, caryophyllene oxide
- α-pinene, β-pinene, γ-terpinene, sabinene, limonene, myrcene, camphene, *p*-cymene, thujene
- α-terpineol, terpinen-4-ol, borneol, linalool, *trans*-pinocarveol, geraniol
- methyl chavicol (estragole)

## BLEND

| 10 drops | *Hyssop* |
| 10 drops | *Juniper Berry* |
| <u>20 drops</u> | *Chamomile Roman* |
| <u>40 drops</u> | *BLEND* |

Make up your *BLEND* using the quantities above – store in a small dark glass bottle fitted with a dropper.

## AILMENT

Bursitis is literally inflammation of the bursa. A bursa is a small sac filled with fluid that lubricates the joints by allowing skin, muscles and tendons to move smoothly over the bones. The inflammation can be bactericidal or due to conditions such as rheumatism. It is nearly always caused by repeated pressure, friction or injury. Names for bursitis attacks such as 'housemaid's knee', 'tennis elbow', 'dustman's shoulder' etc. are still in common use.

In bursitis extra fluid collects around the joint impeding movement and causing heat, swelling and pain.

Arthritis and gout can also give rise to bursitis.

## APPLICATION

To reduce the heat and swelling prepare an ice cold bowl of water and add 5 drops of *BLEND*. Use a cotton cloth to make a compress. Soak the cloth in the prepared water, wring out and apply to the inflamed area.

Another way to cool the area is to freeze a cardboard cup of water – the ice will protrude above the lip of the cup. You can massage this gently over the swollen area.

## MASSAGE

Make up a bottle of Bursitis Treatment Oil by adding 12 drops of *BLEND* to 30 ml of Sweet Almond Oil.

Rub the Treatment Oil gently around the affected area at least twice daily. The oils will penetrate the skin and help to combat the infection. *Juniper Berry* is a diuretic which will help to reduce the swelling.

## BATHS

Add 8 drops of *BLEND* to your bath. Take plenty of time to soak in the bath. The warmth will comfort the pain and the oils will help the infection.

## LIFE STYLE

Once the swelling begins to subside you can exercise the affected joint daily. Exercise for only a minute or two at a time to start with. Repeat this frequently during the day. Avoid any pressure on the joint and avoid any repetitive use of it.

# Cellulite

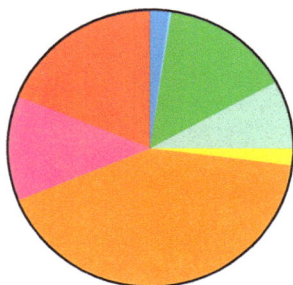

| | | |
|---|---|---|
| | esters | 2.1% |
| | aliphatic aldehydes | |
| | ketones | 0.5% |
| | sesquiterpenes | 14.8% |
| | lactones & coumarins | trace |
| | remainder | 8.0% |
| | oxides | 1.8% |
| | acids | trace |
| | aromatic aldehydes | |
| | monoterpenes | 42.0% |
| | alcohols | 12.1% |
| | phenols, phe. ethers | 18.7% |

**CCP of BLEND RECIPE**

*Juniper Berry* (juniperus communis)

*Cypress* (cupressus sempervirens)

*Patchouli* (pogostemon cablin)

*Oreganum* (origanum vulgaris)

*Juniper Berry* is recommended for breaking down cellulite and removing excess body fluid Avoid in pregnancy and if kidneys are inflamed.

*Cypress* regulates, balances and is a good decongestant. Recommended for cellulite, and rheumatism. Constricts blood vessels and combats excesses.

*Patchouli* is an astringent, decongestant and an excellent oil for encouraging good skin condition.

*Oreganum* a powerful oil that is a diuretic and cleanses the body by causing sweating. Avoid in pregnancy.

*Chemical constituents to be found in the blend may include:*

- linalyl acetate, terpinyl acetate
- patchoulenone, isopatchoulenone
- caryophyllene, cadinene, cedrene, patchoulenes, humulenes, α-guaiene
- 1.8-cineole, manoyl oxide, guaiene-oxide, bulnesene oxide, caryophyllene oxide
- α-pinene, β-pinene, γ-terpinene, α-terpinene, limonene, sabinene, p-cymene, myrcene
- α-terpineol, sabinol, pogostol, patchouli alcohols, manool, linalool, cedrol, guaiol, bulnesol
- carvacrol, thymol

## BLEND

| | |
|---|---|
| 10 drops | *Juniper Berry* |
| 10 drops | *Cypress* |
| 10 drops | *Patchouli* |
| <u>10 drops</u> | *Oreganum* |
| <u>40 drops</u> | *BLEND* |

Make up your *BLEND* using the quantities above – store in a small dark glass bottle fitted with a dropper.

## AILMENT

Research in France, Italy and Germany has revealed that constipation, poor lymphatic system, poor circulation and weak functioning of the kidney and liver are more common in women prone to cellulite. Cellulite shows as lumpy puckered tissue giving the skin an appearance similar to orange peel. It tends to collect on the thighs and buttocks and sometimes on the arms as well. Essential oils can help to break down these fatty deposits and attention to diet will also be beneficial.

## MASSAGE

Make up a bottle of Cellulite Treatment Oil by adding 12 drops of *BLEND* to 30 ml of Sweet Almond Oil.

Massage the Treatment Oil twice daily all around the affected body areas. Use a firm pressure and work in strong circular movements using the palm of your hand. Increase the pressure as you become accustomed to the massage action.

To improve your blood and lymph circulation organise to have regular professional massage treatments.

## BATHS

Add 8 drops of *BLEND* to your bath. Soak well and allow plenty of time for the oils to be absorbed into the body. They will begin to break down the fatty tissues.

## SKIN BRUSHING

Skin brushing will help stimulate the lymph system. Use a long handled natural-bristle hair brush or a friction glove. Friction gloves can be purchased from the chemist. Follow a daily routine – brush the complete body, except for the face, first thing in the morning and last thing at night. Start gently and increase the pressure as the body becomes used to the treatment.

## DIET

Some naturopaths recommend a diet of 75% raw food to prevent the cellulite from forming and to eliminate the existing cells.

Other recommended foods are:

Beetroot juice – good for liver function
Celery – good for excess fluid
Cucumber – good for kidneys
Watermelon – good for excess fluid

General weight loss usually improves the condition considerably.

# Chickenpox

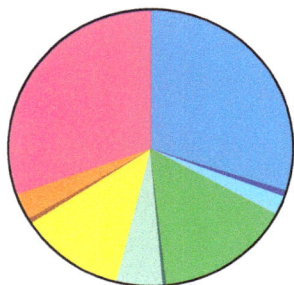

| | | |
|---|---|---|
| 🟦 | esters | 30.0% |
| 🟦 | aliphatic aldehydes | 0.7% |
| 🟦 | ketones | 2.7% |
| 🟩 | sesquiterpenes | 15.0% |
| 🟩 | lactones & coumarins | 0.2% |
| 🟩 | remainder | 4.1% |
| 🟨 | oxides | 13.0% |
| 🟨 | acids | |
| 🟫 | aromatic aldehydes | 0.7% |
| 🟧 | monoterpenes | 3.0% |
| 🟪 | alcohols | 30.6% |
| 🟧 | phenols, phe. ethers | trace |

**CCP of BLEND RECIPE**

*Lavender True* (lavandula angustifolia)

*Chamomile German* (matricaria recutica)

*Lavender True* is excellent for the regeneration of skin cells. It heals wounds and scars and is on the whole a calming oil. It also has analgesic properties and helps with anxiety and migraines. It is recommended for burns, eczema, psoriasis, spots and blisters.

*Chamomile German* is analgesic, antiinflammatory, temperature reducing and hormone like. It is useful for treating acne, boils, burns, insect bites, psoriasis, rheumatism, toothache, wounds and ulcers. This oil is a cooling treatment for the skin. The deep blue colour is due to the chamazulene which forms during distillation.

This blend of two oils will give relief to the itchiness of the patient's skin whilst guarding against infection getting into the chickenpox spots.

*Chemical constituents to be found in the blend may include:*

🟦 linalyl acetate, lavandulyl acetate, geranyl acetate
🟦 citral
🟦 octanone, camphor
🟩 β-caryophyllene, farnesene, chamazulene
🟩 coumarin, umbelliferone

🟩 en-yn-dicycloether, *cis*-spiro-ether
🟨 1.8-cineole, α-bisabolol oxide, linalool oxide, caryophyllene oxide
🟫 cuminaldehyde, benzaldehyde
🟧 ocimene, camphene, limonene
🟪 terpinen-4-ol, α-terpineol, borneol, α-bisabolol, linalool, lavandulol, geraniol

## BLEND

| | |
|---|---|
| 28 drops | *Lavender True* |
| <u>14 drops</u> | *Chamomile German* |
| <u>42 drops</u> | *BLEND* |

Make up your *BLEND* using the quantities above – store in a small dark glass bottle fitted with a dropper.

## AILMENT

A most infectious and common virus. An attack of the chickenpox virus (varicella) often confers lifelong immunity although the virus always remains in the body and can break out again. Because of this immunity it is mainly suffered in childhood. The virus takes about 14 days to incubate and the sufferer is highly infectious 4 days before the rash appears until the final scabs have healed. The rash starts, together with a temperature, as small raised spots which progress into very unsightly inflamed blisters. The spots start on the trunk and spread to the face and limbs. Despite the horrendous appearance of the skin with such ugly blisters the skin usually makes a complete recovery, especially if the patient resists the urge to scratch.

If contracted as an adult the attack is likely to be much more severe and the patient can feel very ill for the first few days.

The same virus is responsible for both shingles and herpes.

An outbreak of shingles can result in ongoing pain for some months.

Medical treatment for shingles should be sought – especially if the infection gets into the eyes.

## TREATMENT

Make up a bottle of Chickenpox Treatment Lotion by adding 20 drops of *BLEND* to 100 ml of Calamine Lotion.

Apply the Treatment Lotion all over the body twice a day. Rest in bed whilst the fever lasts and get as much sleep as possible.

## BATHS

Add 4 drops of *Lavender True* and 1 cup of bicarbonate of soda to your bath. This will help to relieve the itching.

## VAPOURISER

Place 4 drops of *Tea Tree* (melaleuca alternifolia) in a plant spray full of water. Spray the rooms in the house as a help to combat the spread of the infection.

## DIET

Drink raw vegetable and fruit juices, lemon and orange juice in particular. Lemon tea is also refreshing and beneficial.

# Common Cold

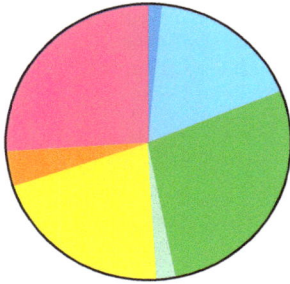

| | | |
|---|---|---|
| | esters | 1.7% |
| | aliphatic aldehydes | trace |
| | ketones | 17.2% |
| | sesquiterpenes | 27.6% |
| | lactones & coumarins | trace |
| | remainder | 2.2% |
| | oxides | 20.8% |
| | acids | trace |
| | aromatic aldehydes | |
| | monoterpenes | 4.0% |
| | alcohols | 26.5% |
| | phenols, phe. ethers | |

**CCP of BLEND RECIPE**

  *Cedarwood Atlas* (cedrus atlantica)

  *Eucalyptus Blue Gum* (eucalyptus globulus)

  *Mint Peppermint* (mentha piperita)

*Cedarwood Atlas* clears mucous and is recommended for bronchitis. It belongs to the Pinaceae family which is generally known for aiding respiratory conditions and is highly antiseptic.

*Eucalyptus Blue Gum* clears nasal passages, reduces temperature and is excellent for all colds.

*Mint Peppermint* lowers fever, is a good expectorant and generally helps mental fatigue.

The blend is well balanced. The ketones and oxides help with the congestion. The alcohols make it highly antiseptic. The sesquiterpenes are calming.

*Chemical constituents to be found in the blend may include:*

| | | |
|---|---|---|
| | atlantone, pinocarvone, menthone | |
| | cadinene, aromadendrene, germac-rene, caryophyllene | |
| | 1.8-cineole | |
| | atlantol, cedrol, globulol, pinocarveol, menthol | |

## BLEND

20 drops   *Cedarwood Atlas*
10 drops   *Eucalyptus Blue Gum*
10 drops   *Mint Peppermint*
40 drops   *BLEND*

Make up your *BLEND* using the quantities above – store in a small dark glass bottle fitted with a dropper.

## GARGLE

A *Tea Tree* oil gargle is helpful at the onset of all colds especially if a sore throat is a symptom.

Add 1 drop of *Tea Tree* (melaleuca alternifolia) oil to a glass of warm boiled water.

Gargle at frequent intervals.

## MASSAGE

Add 12 drops of the *BLEND* to 30 ml of Sweet Almond Oil to make up a supply of Common Cold Treatment Oil.

Alternatively add 12 drops of the *BLEND* to 30 ml of body cream or lotion

Massage chest, neck and upper back areas morning and night.

Concentrate thumb massage around the vertebrae as this stimulates the action of the oils.

A facial massage with this Treatment Oil helps sinusitis sufferers.

Rub a small amount of Treatment Oil under the nostrils when going to bed.

## ROOM SPRAY

Add 12 drops of the *BLEND* to 1 litre of water. Spray freely in any room.

## TISSUES

Place 2 to 4 drops of the *BLEND* onto a paper tissue.

Wrap the tissue in foil and pop it in your pocket so that you can inhale the vapours from the tissue at regular intervals during the day.

To ease congestion at night place such a tissue on the soles of your feet. The vapour from the oils passes around the body as you sleep.

## VAPOURISER

Place 4 to 6 drops of the *BLEND* in the vapouriser.

It helps to keep the vapouriser going in any room where you are spending any length of time.

This also guards against others contracting your condition.

## BATHS

Place 8 drops of the *BLEND* into a warm bath.

Relax and inhale the vapours.

This is particularly helpful before going to bed.

## DIET

Two or three garlic tablets each day are recommended.

Cut down on all dairy food as this encourages the production of mucous in the system.

Take regular doses of vitamin C tablets or drinks.

Follow a light healthy diet of fruit and vegetables.

# Constipation

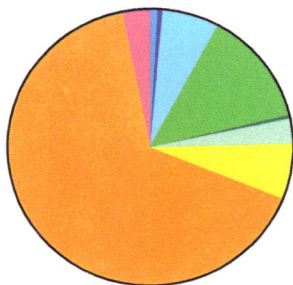

| | | |
|---|---|---|
| ☐ | esters | 1.0% |
| ☐ | aliphatic aldehydes | 0.8% |
| ☐ | ketones | 6.6% |
| ☐ | sesquiterpenes | 12.8% |
| ☐ | lactones & coumarins | 0.2% |
| ☐ | remainder | 3.3% |
| ☐ | oxides | 6.2% |
| ☐ | acids | trace |
| ☐ | aromatic aldehydes | trace |
| ☐ | monoterpenes | 66.0% |
| ☐ | alcohols | 3.1% |
| ☐ | phenols, phe. ethers | trace |

## CCP of BLEND RECIPE

*Orange Bitter* (citrus aurantium amara)

*Black Pepper* (piper nigrum)

*Rosemary* (rosmarinus officinalis)

*Orange Bitter* is a calming cheering oil that is generally helpful to the digestive system. It treats both nervous indigestion and constipation. Also it is a stimulant to the liver.

*Black Pepper* is a warming and stimulating oil. It is extremely helpful to the digestive system, stimulating the liver and pancreas. It is recommended for constipation, flatulence and indigestion and also tones the colon muscles.

*Rosemary* is an antispasmodic and analgesic and stimulates bile production. Traditionally the Greeks and Romans considered it to be a sacred plant bringing peace and comfort. It is a smooth muscle relaxant. Do not use if epilepsy is suspected.

*Chemical constituents to be found in the blend may include:*

☐ linalyl acetate, geranyl acetate, citron-ellyl acetate, bornyl acetate

☐ undecanal, citral

☐ piperitone, dihydrocarvone, camphor, carvone, thujone

☐ β-caryophyllene, bisabolene, humu-lenes, farnesene, copaene

☐ caryophyllene oxide, 1.8-cineole

☐ piperonal

☐ limonene, α-pinene, myrcene, β-pinene, sabinene, camphene, *p*-cymene, phellandrene, ocimene

☐ linalool, nerol, α-terpineol, citronellol, terpinen-4-ol, borneol

## BLEND

| 16 drops | *Orange Bitter* |
|---|---|
| 16 drops | *Black Pepper* |
| 8 drops | *Rosemary* |
| 40 drops | *BLEND* |

Make up your *BLEND* using the quantities above – store in a small dark glass bottle fitted with a dropper.

## AILMENT

Constipation, strictly speaking, is a symptom rather than an ailment. It is an indication that for some reason the body is not able to function as it should. Life style, diet and each person's constitution affect bowel habits. It is quite normal for some people to have 3 bowel actions a day and quite normal for other people to have a bowel movement just 3 times a week. Irregular and frequent small hard motions are the signs of constipation problems looming.

## MASSAGE

Make up a bottle of Constipation Treatment Oil by adding 12 drops of *BLEND* to 30 ml of Sweet Almond Oil.

Rub the oil all over the abdomen. Cover the whole area starting at the hair line and working up to the chest. Use gentle circular strokes.

You can gently rub a little of the Treatment Oil around and just inside the anus the encourage the intestinal reflex to work.

## LIFE STYLE

A readily identifiable cause of constipation is the taking of drugs. Morphine and its derivatives such as codeine are almost certain to have constipation as a side effect. Some drugs for lowering blood pressure and some anti-depressants are equally guilty.

Failure of the intestinal reflexes as a result of old age is common and chronic. It then becomes necessary to take gentle laxatives to deal with the problem. However in general do not resort to purges or strong laxatives as they can set up a vicious circle of events.

Take regular exercise to condition your stomach and back muscles this can in turn aid the bowel movements. Visit the lavatory at regular intervals – take a good book and relax allowing the body to resume its regular habits.

## DIET

Drink at least 8 glasses of mineral water a day. Good natural laxatives are broccoli, cabbage, prunes and figs. Bran is also recommended and in general stick to a diet that includes plenty of fluid and fibre.

# Cramp

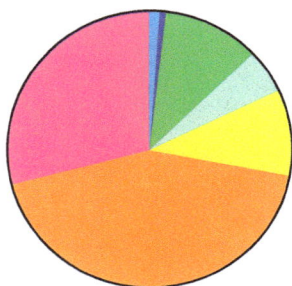

| | | |
|---|---|---|
| 🟦 | esters | 1.1% |
| 🟦 | aliphatic aldehydes | 0.7% |
| 🟦 | ketones | |
| 🟩 | sesquiterpenes | 11.3% |
| 🟩 | lactones & coumarins | trace |
| ⬜ | remainder | 5.1% |
| 🟨 | oxides | 10.0% |
| 🟨 | acids | |
| 🟫 | aromatic aldehydes | |
| 🟧 | monoterpenes | 43.1% |
| 🟪 | alcohols | 28.7% |
| 🟧 | phenols, phe. ethers | trace |

**CCP of BLEND RECIPE**

🔴 💧💧💧 *Marjoram Sweet* (origanum majorana)

🟠 💧💧 *Mandarin* (citrus reticulata)

🟡 💧💧 *Chamomile German* (matricaria recutica)

*Marjoram Sweet* is analgesic, antispasmodic, balancing and calming. It helps circulation and is vasodilatory. Used for treating muscle aches, bruising, cramps and rheumatism. Known in folk lore as 'joy of the mountain'.

*Mandarin* is antispasmodic and revitalising offering help for anxiety and stress. Balances metabolic rate. This fruit was given to the Mandarins as a mark of respect.

*Chamomile German* is again an antispasmodic oil. It calms the system down and helps with back pain and any muscular spasms. Good for intestinal colic and flatulence.

### Chemical constituents to be found in the blend may include:

🟦 linalyl acetate, terpinyl acetate, geranyl acetate, methyl anthranilate
🟦 citral, citronellal
🟩 caryophyllene, cadinene, chamazulene, farnesene
⬜ en-yn-dicycloether, *cis*-spiro ether
🟨 α-bisabolol oxide
🟧 β-pinene, α-terpinene, γ-terpinene, *p*-cymene, myrcene, limonene, ocimene, sabinene
🟪 linalool, borneol, α-terpineol, terpin-en-4-ol, α-bisabolol
🟧 carvacrol, eugenol, thymol

## BLEND

| | |
|---|---|
| 18 drops | *Marjoram Sweet* |
| 12 drops | *Mandarin* |
| 12 drops | *Chamomile German* |
| 42 drops | *BLEND* |

Make up your *BLEND* using the quantities above – store in a small dark glass bottle fitted with a dropper.

## AILMENT

Cramp is a painful spasm of a muscle – very often suffered in a calf or thigh muscle. The muscles contract involuntarily and suddenly causing severe pain. The contraction can last for several minutes. Even the bravest of people cry out at such pain. The known causes for these muscle contractions to be triggered involuntarily are a shortage of salts in the system, due maybe to excessive sweating, or bodily fatigue or a deficient blood supply due to poor circulation.

## FIRST AID

To relieve the cramp it is necessary to stretch the cramped muscles.

If the thigh muscles are cramped sit down, straighten out the leg and get a helper to lift the foot in one hand whilst pushing firmly down on the knee with the other hand.

Another possible way to break the contraction is to press firmly on the nail of the big toe and apply strong pressure to both the front and the back of the toe.

For hand cramp force the fingers apart and place the finger tips firmly down on a cold surface.

## MASSAGE

Make up a bottle of Cramp Treatment Oil by adding 12 drops of *BLEND* to 30 ml of Sweet Almond Oil.

Massage gently around the muscle area as soon as the cramp has subsided.

Before going to bed at night massage the whole leg upwards with the Treatment Oil.

Also massage the Treatment Oil well into your feet. It is most important that your feet are warm and that the blood is circulating to them. Put warm bed socks on and place a soft pillow beneath your feet. In this way your feet will remain warm throughout the night.

## BATHS

Add 8 drops of *BLEND* to your baths.

## DIET

If the cause of your cramp attacks is poor circulation follow a low fat diet to ensure that your cholesterol level is kept low.

If the cause is due to lack of salts in the blood then increase your intake of salt for a while to restore the balance.

**Supplements**

Multi vitamin/mineral tablet
B Complex as per container
Vitamin C 1000 mgs a day
Garlic capsules as per container
Evening Primrose Oil – 2 tablets daily.

# Cystitis

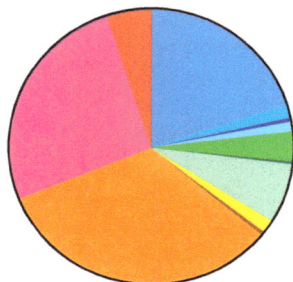

| | | |
|---|---|---|
| ■ | esters | 20.6% |
| ■ | aliphatic aldehydes | 0.4% |
| ■ | ketones | 1.6% |
| ■ | sesquiterpenes | 4.2% |
| ■ | lactones & coumarins | 0.1% |
| ■ | remainder | 7.1% |
| ■ | oxides | 1.6% |
| ■ | acids | trace |
| ■ | aromatic aldehydes | 0.4% |
| ■ | monoterpenes | 32.6% |
| ■ | alcohols | 26.4% |
| ■ | phenols, phe. ethers | 5.0% |

## CCP of BLEND RECIPE

*Basil Sweet European* (ocimum basilicum)

*Lavender True* (lavandula angustifolia)

*Pine Scotch* (pinus sylvestris)

*Basil Sweet European* is antiviral, bactericidal. It is a stimulant and tonic having a strong cleansing effect on the body. It cleanses the kidneys, helps with congested prostate and attacks cistitis.

*Lavender True* is a calming gentle oil and is strongly bactericidal. It not only clears infections it also helps sore and damaged skin to heal quickly.

*Pine Scotch* is antiinflammatory antiseptic. It has a hormone like action and brings the body back to balance. It has a fresh forest like aroma. It is acknowledged that pine forests produce a healing environment due to evaporation of the essential oil from the pine needles.

### *Chemical constituents to be found in the blend may include:*

- ■ linalyl acetate, fenchyl acetate, methyl cinnamate, lavandulyl acetate, bornyl acetate, terpinyl acetate
- ■ citronellal, citral
- ■ octanone, camphor, cryptone
- ■ β-caryophyllene, cadinene, copaene, guaiene, farnesene
- ■ coumarin, umbelliferone

- ■ 1.8-cineole, linalool oxide
- ■ cuminaldehyde, benzaldehyde
- ■ *cis*-ocimene, α-pinene, β-pinene, limonene, myrcene, sabinene
- ■ α-terpineol, linalool, borneol, lavandulol, terpinen-4-ol
- ■ eugenol, methyl chavicol

## BLEND

| 8 drops | *Basil Sweet European* |
| 16 drops | *Lavender True* |
| <u>16 drops</u> | *Pine Scotch* |
| <u>40 drops</u> | *BLEND* |

Make up your *BLEND* using the quantities above – store in a small dark glass bottle fitted with a dropper.

## AILMENT

Cystitis causes a burning pain on passing urine and urges frequent trips to the lavatory to find it is only possible to pass a few drops. Also the sufferer can fell quite unwell in themselves.

Cystitis is an inflamed membrane in the bowel usually caused by bacterial infection that has travelled up the urinary passage. Due to the fact that this passage is much shorter in women than in men women are the main sufferers of this condition. It can also be triggered by food allergy, chemical sensitivity, bruising during intercourse and vaginal thrush.

It can clear up within hours or may develop into a life long problem.

If blood appears in the urine seek medical advice.

## TREATMENT

Make up a bottle of Cystitis Treatment Oil by adding 12 drops of *BLEND* to 30 ml of Sweet Almond Oil.

Use this soothing Treatment Oil and apply to gently to the entrance to the urinal passage. Do this 2 or 3 times a day.

Once a day lie quietly and massage this Treatment Oil over the abdomen, hips and lower back.

Help your body combat the infection by taking plenty of rest if necessary take some bed rest.

## BATHS

Add 8 drops of *BLEND* to your bath. Take 2 or 3 baths a day soak for at least 10 to 15 minutes. This will help you to deal with the discomfort.

## DIET

Drink at least 8 glasses of spring water a day.

Until the condition clears avoid, as far as possible, all acid producing foods such as:

citrus or sour fruits,
vinegars,
animal proteins such as eggs, fish, meat and cheese.

# Diarrhoea

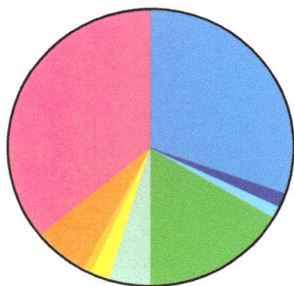

| | | |
|---|---|---|
| ■ | esters | 30.4% |
| ■ | aliphatic aldehydes | 1.8% |
| ■ | ketones | 1.6% |
| ■ | sesquiterpenes | 16.2% |
| ■ | lactones & coumarins | trace |
| ■ | remainder | 4.7% |
| ■ | oxides | 2.3% |
| ■ | acids | 1.0% |
| ■ | aromatic aldehydes | |
| ■ | monoterpenes | 6.0% |
| ■ | alcohols | 36.0% |
| ■ | phenols, phe. ethers | trace |

## CCP of BLEND RECIPE

 💧 *Ginger* (zingiber officinale)

 💧💧 *Sandalwood* (santalum album)

 💧💧 *Chamomile Roman* (chamaemelum nobile)

*Ginger* is antispasmodic and temperature reducing. Its warm spicy aroma is comforting. Excellent oil for all digestive upsets. Used in many ancient recipes.

*Sandalwood* has a musty lingering aroma that creates a feeling of peace. It is a sedative and calming oil.

*Chamomile Roman* helpful for intestinal colic. It is antispasmodic, calming and sedative and also reduces temperature and fever. This oil is highly respected for its calming influence on all systems. Known as the plant's physician as it protects neighbouring plants from infections.

### *Chemical constituents to be found in the blend may include:*

■ angelates, tiglates, butyrates, propionates
■ geranial, citronellals
■ gingerone, santalone, pinocarvone
■ β-sesquiphellandrene, zingiberene, santalenes, curcumenes, farnesene, chamazulene, caryophyllene

■ 1.8-cineole
■ nortricycloekasantalic acid
■ α-pinene, β-pinene, camphene, limonene, phellandrene, sabinene
■ citronellol, linalool, borneol, gingerol, santalols, tricycloekasantalol, farnesol, nerolidol, α-terpineol, *trans*-pinocarveol

## BLEND

| 8 drops | *Ginger* |
|---|---|
| 16 drops | *Sandalwood* |
| <u>16 drops</u> | *Chamomile Roman* |
| <u>40 drops</u> | *BLEND* |

Make up your *BLEND* using the quantities above – store in a small dark glass bottle fitted with a dropper.

## AILMENT

Most diarrhoea is due to inflammation of the intestines. This inflammation is commonly caused by viruses, bacterial food poisoning or less commonly by larger parasites such as amoebic dysentery or worms.

Nervous upset can also cause the condition as disturbances of the endocrine hormonal output can over activate the intestinal action.

Irritable colon, a common complaint, is often the result of anxiety and sometimes made worse by constant taking of laxatives. Laxatives can irritate the colon and cause it to form too much mucous which is then mistaken for diarrhoea.

If the diarrhoea persists without relief for 2 to 3 days seek medical advice.

## PREVENTION

Always make sure that food is thoroughly washed and clean. Take extra precautions if travelling and only drink bottled water.

Establish a regular pattern of eating wholesome foods and try to establish a regular bowel action. Try to reduce stress levels.

## MASSAGE

Make up a bottle of Diarrhoea Treatment Oil by adding 12 drops of *BLEND* to 30 ml of Sweet Almond Oil.

Massage your abdomen and lower back. Work with gentle circular stokes in a clockwise direction. Repeat the treatment every 2 to 3 hours whilst the condition persists. Take time to relax and unwind.

## BATHS

Add 8 drops of *BLEND* to your bath. Take time to relax and the essential oils will help to balance your system.

## DIET

It is very important not to become dehydrated during an attack of diarrhoea. The body loses salts faster than it can replace them. Make a replacement drink by preparing a glass of warm water to which you add some sugar and a pinch of salt. Take frequent small drinks of this. It is also possible to buy sachets of prepared minerals from the chemist if you prefer.

Another drink that often settles an upset stomach is a glass of warm water with one teaspoon of honey and one drop of *Mint Peppermint* (mentha piperita) Again sip it gradually.

Avoid all foods that are likely to create acid levels as these will prompt the intestine to produce too much mucous.

It is a good idea to fast for several hours and then gradually introduce bland foods. This helps the system to recover.

# Eczema

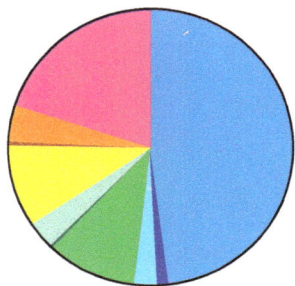

| | | |
|---|---|---|
| 🟦 | esters | 48.0% |
| 🟦 | aliphatic aldehydes | 1.2% |
| 🟦 | ketones | 2.8% |
| 🟩 | sesquiterpenes | 10.2% |
| 🟩 | lactones & coumarins | 0.1% |
| 🟦 | remainder | 3.3% |
| 🟨 | oxides | 9.8% |
| 🟨 | acids | trace |
| 🟫 | aromatic aldehydes | 0.4% |
| 🟧 | monoterpenes | 3.8% |
| 🟥 | alcohols | 20.4% |
| 🟧 | phenols, phe. ethers | trace |

## CCP of BLEND RECIPE

 🌢🌢 *Chamomile Roman* (chamaemelum nobile)

 🌢🌢 *Lavender True* (lavandula angustifolia)

 🌢 *Chamomile German* (matricaria recutica)

*Chamomile Roman* has a very cooling effect on the skin and calms all the body systems down. It is excellent for easing the irritation caused by eczema.

*Lavender True* helps to heal skin wounds and keeps infection at bay. Its beautiful aroma is also very soothing.

*Chamomile German* is good for all states of tension and nervous reaction to stress. This oil is recommended for acne, allergies, boils, burns, psoriasis, rashes, ulcers and wounds. It has a warm herby aroma.

---

*Chemical constituents to be found in the blend may include:*

🟦 angelates, tiglates, linalyl acetate, geranyl acetate, lavandulyl acetate
🟦 citral
🟦 pinocarvone, octanone, camphor
🟩 chamazulene, β-caryophyllene, farnesene
🟩 coumarin, umbelliferone

🟦 en-yn-dicycloether, *cis*-spiro-ether
🟨 α-bisabolol oxide. 1.8-cineole, caryophyllene oxide, linalool oxide
🟫 cuminaldehyde, benzaldehyde
🟥 α-bisabolol, farnesol, nerolidol, α-terpineol, trans-pinocarveol, terpinen-4-ol, linalool, borneol, geraniol, lavandulol

## BLEND

| | |
|---|---|
| 16 drops | *Chamomile Roman* |
| 16 drops | *Lavender True* |
| 8 drops | *Chamomile German* |
| 40 drops | *BLEND* |

Make up your *BLEND* using the quantities above – store in a small dark glass bottle fitted with a dropper.

## AILMENT

Eczema appears as an inflamed area of skin which is extremely itchy. It often develops into blisters that weep and form crusty scabs.

There are two types of eczema. The first called contact eczema appears within minutes of contact with substances that cause the skin to react. The substances can be as diverse as gold and wax polish. The second type of eczema called atopic eczema is much more difficult to deal with. In this case the cause is difficult to track down. Very often people prone to these inexplicable attacks of eczema are allergy sufferers. It is also believed that extreme unhappiness or life stress can prompt outbreaks of eczema. Eczema in young children tends to gradually diminish as they grow up.

Unfortunately for adult atopic eczema sufferers it can take a long time to discover the cause.

## APPLICATION

Make up a bottle of Eczema Treatment Oil by adding 12 drops of *BLEND* to 30 ml of Sweet Almond Oil.

To help with the discomfort apply the Treatment Oil to the affected areas night and morning.

If the irritation is very bad during the day make up a pot of eczema Treatment Lotion by adding 12 drops of *BLEND* to 30 ml of lotion. Apply the lotion gently to the area.

Try to overcome the urge to scratch at all times as it will only irritate the skin further. Just placing your hand firmly over the irritating area may help you to cope.

## BATHS

Add 8 drops of *BLEND* to your bath. Make sure the water temperature is not too hot. Taking a bath can really help to cope with the irritation.

## LIFE STYLE

If you suspect the eczema attack may be linked to personal stress and emotional upset you must try to resolve your situation. It may be advisable to seek some professional counselling. A useful address for eczema sufferers is:

National Eczema Society, Tavistock House, Tavistock Square, London, WC1.

## DIET

If you suspect that your eczema attack is due to food allergy then devise a method for tracking down the guilty party. Start by restricting your diet to just a few items. If that is successful just add an extra item at a time. Professional consultants can help you set up such a programme.

# **Emotional Stress**

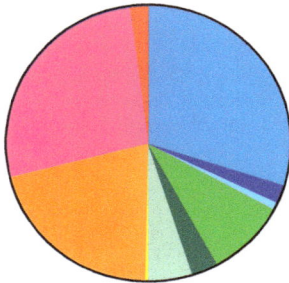

| | | |
|---|---|---|
| 🟦 | esters | 30.0% |
| 🟪 | aliphatic aldehydes | 1.6% |
| 🟦 | ketones | 1.4% |
| 🟩 | sesquiterpenes | 9.1% |
| 🟩 | lactones & coumarins | 3.0% |
| 🟩 | remainder | 4.8% |
| 🟨 | oxides | 0.4% |
| 🟨 | acids | trace |
| 🟫 | aromatic aldehydes | |
| 🟧 | monoterpenes | 20.3% |
| 🟥 | alcohols | 27.4% |
| 🟧 | phenols, phe. ethers | 2.0% |

**CCP of BLEND RECIPE**

*Geranium* (pelargonium graveolens)

*Bergamot* (citrus bergamia)

*Ylang Ylang* (cananga odorata)

*Geranium* is an excellent all round balancer, eliminates waste and congestion. It calms nervous fatigue and regulates hormonal function.

*Bergamot* calms anxiety. It also assists skin to heal. It can be most helpful at combating depression. It encourages confidence and revitalises.

*Ylang Ylang* helps with anxiety, fear, depression and panic. It slows the breathing pace. It has a sweet heavy exotic aroma.

The largest chemical families in this blend are the esters, sesquiterpenes, monoterpenes and alcohols. Thus the blend shows a good balance between calming and cheering aspects.

*Chemical constituents to be found in the blend may include:*

🟦 linalyl acetate, citronellyl acetate, benzyl acetate, geranyl acetate
🟪 citral
🟦 menthone
🟩 β-caryophyllene, germacrene, β-bisabolene, guaiazulene

🟩 bergaptene
🟨 *cis*-rose oxide
🟧 α-pinene, β-pinene, γ-terpinene, limonene, α-terpinene
🟥 linalool, farnesol, geraniol, citronellol
🟧 eugenol, safrole

## BLEND

| 8 drops | *Geranium* |
| 24 drops | *Bergamot* |
| 8 drops | *Ylang Ylang* |
| 40 drops | *BLEND* |

Make up your *BLEND* using the quantities above – store in a small dark glass bottle fitted with a dropper.

## MASSAGE

Make up a bottle of Emotional Stress Treatment Oil by adding 12 drops of *BLEND* to 30 ml of Sweet Almond Oil.

Take time to sit quietly and massage your feet and hands with this Treatment Oil.

If possible ask a friend or partner to give you a soothing shoulder massage. A great deal of tension is held in the shoulders and neck.

Emotional stress is a condition that is greatly helped by visiting a professional aromatherapist at regular intervals. Weekly visits to start with can prove extremely helpful.

## RELAXATION

It is vital to find time to relax. Make time during the day to sit quietly in peaceful surroundings.

Taking tuition in the Alexander Technique can be beneficial. Many people with demanding work find this helpful.

## ANXIETY ATTACKS

Many people suffering from emotional stress are liable to panic attacks. For immediate relief put 3 drops of *Bergamot* oil onto a tissue and inhale gently. If you are prone to such attacks carry a tissue with you.

## LIFE STYLE

Take gentle walks, attend relaxation sessions such as Alexander Technique and Yoga. Daily swimming is also excellent for helping the body relax.

## DIET

Follow a light healthy diet of fruit and vegetables. Cut out any heavy fatty foods.

Avoid strong stimulants such as coffee and tea.

## OTHER ESSENTIAL OILS

Other oils that can be helpful during times of emotional stress are:

*Palma Rosa, Lavender True, Juniper Berry, Sweet Marjoram, Rose and Sandalwood.*

# Fluid Retention

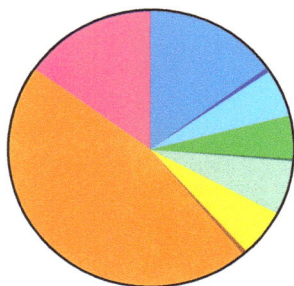

| | | |
|---|---|---|
| ■ | esters | 15.2% |
| ■ | aliphatic aldehydes | 0.3% |
| ■ | ketones | 5.5% |
| ■ | sesquiterpenes | 5.2% |
| ■ | lactones & coumarins | 0.1% |
| ■ | remainder | 6.4% |
| ■ | oxides | 5.7% |
| ■ | acids | trace |
| ■ | aromatic aldehydes | 0.3% |
| ■ | monoterpenes | 46.3% |
| ■ | alcohols | 15.0% |
| ■ | phenols, phe. ethers | trace |

**CCP of BLEND RECIPE**

*Juniper Berry* (juniperus communis)

*Lavender True* (lavandula angustifolia)

*Rosemary* (rosmarinus officinalis)

*Juniper Berry* is excellent for cleansing the body. It is recommended for cellulite, fluid retention, obesity, clearing fluid from oedemas and eliminating uric acid from painful joints.

*Lavender True* is antiinflammatory and antiseptic. It is excellent for helping skin conditions and is a generally balancing oil.

*Rosemary* is a stimulating oil. It is a diuretic and a decongestant. It stimulates the memory and helps with fatigue and depression.

*Chemical constituents to be found in the blend may include:*

■ linalyl acetate, geranyl acetate, lavandulyl acetate, fenchyl acetate, bornyl acetate, terpinyl acetate
■ citral
■ camphor, carvone, thujone, octanone
■ β-caryophyllene, cadinene, humulenes, germacrene
■ coumarin, umbelliferone

■ 1.8-cineole, linalool oxide, caryophyllene oxide
■ cuminaldehyde, benzaldehyde
■ α-pinene, γ-terpinene, myrcene, limonene, sabinene, p-cymene, camphene, ocimene, thujene
■ terpinen-4-ol, α-terpineol, linalool, borneol, geraniol, lavandulol

## BLEND

| 21 drops | *Juniper Berry* |
|----------|-----------------|
| 14 drops | *Lavender True* |
| 7 drops  | *Rosemary*      |
| 42 drops | *BLEND*         |

Make up your *BLEND* using the quantities above – store in a small dark glass bottle fitted with a dropper.

## AILMENT

Fluid retention, known medically as oedema, is the build up of water in the body's fluid tissue to an abnormal level. The body is 60% water which means that an average body has 40 litres of water to be distributed. For this average body to be healthy it needs 3 litres of this water in its blood, 25 litres of this water in its cells and 12 litres of this water in the fluid that the cells are immersed in, called the body's fluid tissue.

Water passes out of the blood in the capillaries into the body's fluid tissue as the pressure from the heart pumping reaches it.

Water passes from the body's fluid tissue back into the blood in the capillaries drawn back by the level of protein in the blood.

Water passes from the blood in the capillaries to the body's tissue fluid drawn out by the level of salt in the body's tissue fluid.

Thus if the pressure from the heart beat is not correct or the level of protein in the blood is not correct or the level of salt in the body tissue fluid is not correct the distribution of the water in the body becomes unbalanced. The amount of water in the body's fluid tissue becomes too much and a swelling results.

If the capillaries become damaged through such things as injury, surgery, burning etc. they can no longer control the balance of this water flow and the tissue swells as the excess is unable to pass back into the blood stream.

## TREATMENT

If the cause of the fluid retention is due the fact that there is too much salt in the body tissue this can be helped by diuretic action. Juniper Berry and Rosemary will help in this case. Fluid retention occurs if you stand for long periods or remain sitting on long journeys. This because the veins are working against gravity and pressure builds on the capillaries. This will right itself when you can move naturally.

## MASSAGE

Make up a bottle of Fluid Retention Treatment Oil by adding 12 drops of *BLEND* to 30 ml of Sweet Almond Oil.

Massage back of legs, lower back and abdomen. The endocrine glands also affect the balance of the water held in the body tissue. This can cause fluid retention to occur during menstruation. Start to use this massage 2 to 3 days before a period.

## DIET

Reducing salt in your diet may be helpful if the retention is caused by too much salt in the system.

Fluid retention in the body tissue is not closely linked to the amount of fluid you drink so cutting this down is not a solution.

# Foot Care

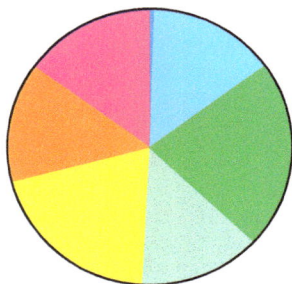

| | | |
|---|---|---|
| 🟦 | esters | 0.4% |
| 🟦 | aliphatic aldehydes | |
| 🟦 | ketones | 14.3% |
| 🟩 | sesquiterpenes | 22.3% |
| 🟩 | lactones & coumarins | trace |
| 🟩 | remainder | 14.1% |
| 🟨 | oxides | 20.0% |
| 🟨 | acids | trace |
| 🟫 | aromatic aldehydes | |
| 🟧 | monoterpenes | 13.7% |
| 🟥 | alcohols | 15.2% |
| 🟧 | phenols, phe. ethers | trace |

**CCP of BLEND RECIPE**

*Tagetes* (tagetes glandulifera)

*Carrot Seed* (daucus carota)

*Chamomile German* (matricaria recutica)

*Tagetes* is antifungal, antiinflammatory, antiseptic and helps skin infections to clear. It is recommended for athlete's foot, bunions, callouses, corns. It has a strong marigold aroma. The tagetes plant is often planted in the vegetable garden to keep pests at bay.

*Carrot Seed* acts in a hormonal way regulating body functions. It is recognised as an antiaging agent and is used to treat chilblains, gout and skin wounds.

*Chamomile German* is a generally soothing oil that has a calming effect on all nervous tensions. It is particular useful in tackling allergic skin reactions.

*Chemical constituents to be found in the blend may include:*

- 🟦 geranyl acetate
- 🟦 citral
- 🟦 tagetone, tagetenones, carvone
- 🟩 daucene, bisabolene, elemene, caryophyllene, chamazulene, farnesene
- 🟩 en-yn-dicycloether, *cis*-spiro-ether
- 🟨 α-bisabolol oxide
- 🟨 valeric acid
- 🟫 salicylaldehyde
- 🟧 limonene, α-pinene, β-pinene, myrcene, camphene
- 🟥 α-bisabolol, linalool
- 🟧 asarone

## BLEND

| 12 drops | *Tagetes* |
|---|---|
| 6 drops | *Carrot Seed* |
| <u>24 drops</u> | *Chamomile German* |
| <u>42 drops</u> | *BLEND* |

Make up your *BLEND* using the quantities above – store in a small dark glass bottle fitted with a dropper.

## FOOT CARE

Our feet are incredibly important to our general well being. The natural massage of the sole of the feet during walking stimulates all the pressure points and the muscle action in the legs keeps our circulation level up.

Healthy well cared for feet can be the basis of a happy life.

## GENERAL CARE

Make up a bottle of Foot Care Treatment Oil by adding 4 drops of *BLEND* to 30 ml of Sweet Almond Oil.

Whenever possible use a little of this Treatment Oil and treat your feet to a relaxing massage with it. Better still get a friend to do it for you. You will find this extraordinarily beneficial.

## FOOT BATH

After a tiring day prepare a warm foot bath by putting 4 drops of *BLEND* in the bowl of water. Relax and soak your feet well.

## BLISTERS

As soon as a blister appears put 1 drop of *Lavender True* and 1 drop of *Tea Tree* directly onto it. If the blister has not burst this will cause the fluid to clear, if it has already burst the oils will heal the wound and protect it from infection.

## CORNS

Make up a bottle of Corn Treatment Oil by adding 1 drops of *Tagetes* to 30 ml of Sweet Almond Oil. Use this to massage your feet from time to time – it will help to prevent corns from forming.

## BUNIONS

Massage around the bunion with the Foot Care Treatment Oil 3 times daily.

## LIFE STYLE

Always cherish your feet. Make sure that all your footwear fits well and is comfortable to walk in. Spend some time walking around barefooted.

If your feet have problems such as ingrowing toe nails or painful corns visit a qualified chiropodist and get expert advice and treatment.

# Gastric Flatulence

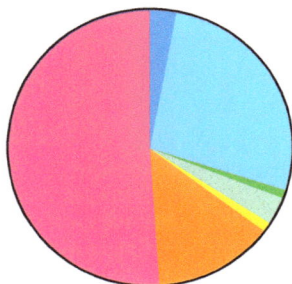

| | | |
|---|---|---|
| | esters | 3.2% |
| | aliphatic aldehydes | trace |
| | ketones | 26.8% |
| | sesquiterpenes | 1.2% |
| | lactones & coumarins | trace |
| | remainder | 3.3% |
| | oxides | 0.9% |
| | acids | trace |
| | aromatic aldehydes | |
| | monoterpenes | 13.8% |
| | alcohols | 50.8% |
| | phenols, phe. ethers | trace |

**CCP of BLEND RECIPE**

 *Coriander* (coriandrum sativum)

 *Mint Spearmint* (mentha spicata)

*Coriander* is a tonic to the digestive system. It is analgesic, antispasmodic, hormone like and will help with mental fatigue and sadness. For the digestive system it will help with anorexia, colic, bad breath, enteritis and indigestion. The aroma is sweet spicy and woody. The herb has been used since ancient times as a herb of happiness – it is used in Benedictine and Chartreuse liqueurs.

*Mint Spearmint* is a digestive tonic and is recommended for bile flow, dyspepsia, flatulence, liver, vomiting. The aroma is spicy warm and minty. Avoid in pregnancy and do not use with young children.

Valued highly as a culinary herb. The water from distillation is used to relieve coughs, colic, hiccoughs and flatulence.

*Chemical constituents to be found in the blend may include:*

- cis-carvyl acetate, linalyl acetate
- decyl aldehyde
- camphor, carvone, menthone
- elemene, farnesene, bourbonene, caryophyllene
- umbelliferone, bergaptene
- 1.8-cineole
- α-pinene, α-terpinene, γ-terpinene, limonene, β-pinene, phellandrene, camphene
- linalool, α-terpineol, geraniol, menthol, borneol
- anethole

## BLEND

24 drops  *Coriander*
16 drops  *Mint Spearmint*
40 drops  *BLEND*

Make up your *BLEND* using the quantities above – store in a small dark glass bottle fitted with a dropper.

## AILMENT

When gas collects in the intestines it can inflict a great deal of discomfort. The flatulence can be caused by swallowing air by eating too quickly. Also if you are tensed up the digestive system can be affected in this way. Further flatulence can build up in the lower part of the intestine due to the fermentation of food.

Sometimes the pressure builds up to such an extent that the swelling can push up into the rib cage. In such a case shortness of breath can be experienced and also angina like pains.

Less commonly, flatulence can be the result of gall stones or the gall bladder being under par.

Should your digestion become really troublesome and also accompanied by weight loss then seek medical advice.

## BATHS

Add 8 drops of *BLEND* to your bath. Allow plenty of time to soak and let the tension relax.

## MASSAGE

Make up a bottle of Gastric Flatulence Treatment Oil by adding 12 drops of *BLEND* to 30 ml of Sweet Almond Oil.

Massage the whole of the abdomen to ease the discomfort. Use gentle circular strokes.

## VAPOURISER

Place 5 drops of *BLEND* in your vapouriser and let the molecules circulate in the room.

## LIFE STYLE

Organise if possible for meal times to be peaceful. Eat slowly. Avoid belching as that also traps air in the stomach.

## DIET

Foods that are likely to cause flatulence are the starchy cellulose foods such as wheat, peas, onions and potatoes etc.

## DRINKS

Prepare a glass of warm water with a teaspoon of honey and 1 drop of *Mint Peppermint* (mentha piperita). Sip slowly.

# Gout

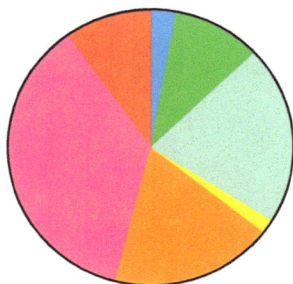

| | |
|---|---|
| esters | 3.0% |
| aliphatic aldehydes | |
| ketones | |
| sesquiterpenes | 10.0% |
| lactones & coumarins | |
| remainder | 20.6% |
| oxides | 1.6% |
| acids | trace |
| aromatic aldehydes | |
| monoterpenes | 19.2% |
| alcohols | 35.6% |
| phenols, phe. ethers | 10.0% |

**CCP of BLEND RECIPE**

 *Basil Sweet European* (ocimum basilicum)

 *Carrot Seed* (daucus carota)

*Basil Sweet European* is antifungal, antiseptic, antiviral and bactericidal. It helps with allergies, gout, acne and reduces the uric acid in the system. The aroma is clear, spicy and sweet. This oil is used extensively in Ayurvedic medicine.

*Carrot Seed* is antiaging, a decongestant. It has a balancing effect on the body and helps to regulate the functions. It dilates blood vessels and is an immune stimulant. It is a diuretic and recommended for gout.

This oil has a dry sweet aroma. It is excellent for general health and well being. Widely used in food flavouring.

*Chemical constituents to be found in the blend may include:*

- linalyl acetate, fenchyl acetate, methyl cinnamate, geranyl acetate
- β-caryophyllene, daucene, elemene, bisabolene
- 1.8-cineole
- α-pinene, β-pinene, γ-terpinene, limonene, *cis*-ocimene, *p*-cymene, camphene
- terpinen-4-ol, α-terpineol, linalool, citronellol, geraniol, carotol, daucol
- methyl chavicol, eugenol, asarone, methyl eugenol

## BLEND

16 drops  *Basil Sweet European*
<u>24 drops</u>  *Carrot Seed*
<u>40 drops</u>  *BLEND*

Make up your *BLEND* using the quantities above – store in a small dark glass bottle fitted with a dropper.

## AILMENT

Gout is the build up of uric acid that forms crystals around the joints.

Although all foods are a potential source of uric acid they are not normally the main culprit. The body synthesis should maintain the correct levels of uric acid in the tissues, however over synthesis can result in the uric acid crystals being deposited. Thus this ailment is likely to be due to hereditary biochemical problems.

Attacks of gout appear without warning – a single joint is suddenly inflamed and extremely painful. The uric acid crystals are seen by the body as 'foreign bodies'.

Unfortunately the immune system attacks and in a sense attacks the body itself. Grumbling arthritis is also a form of gout.

It can become a dangerous condition if the uric acid crystals form in the kidneys.

## BATHS

Put 8 drops of *BLEND* in your bath water. Soak well, the warmth eases the pain.

## MASSAGE

Make up a bottle of Gout Treatment Oil by adding 12 drops of *BLEND* to 30 ml of Sweet Almond Oil.

Massage the Treatment Oil near to the inflamed joint but not actually on it. Get a friend to give you a back massage as this will allow the oils to enter the blood stream and travel to the affected area.

## COMPRESSES

Prepare a bowl of warm water add 4 drops of *BLEND*. Use a cotton cloth to make a compress. Soak the cloth in the prepared water, wring out and wrap around the affected joint.

## FOOT BATHS

If the feet are affected treat them to frequent foot baths. Prepare a bowl of warm water and add 4 drops of *BLEND*. Soak the feet well in the prepared water.

## DIET

Foods high in uric acid are liver and kidneys.

Cut back on red meats, dairy produce and alcohol. Concentrate on fish and green vegetables.

**Daily Supplements**
Vitamin C    1000 mgs
Vitamin E    250 mgs
One teaspoon of Codliver Oil plus 5 drops of Evening Primrose Oil.

# Haemorrhoids

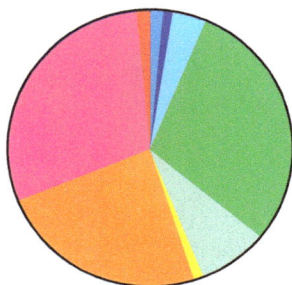

| | | |
|---|---|---|
| | esters | 1.6% |
| | aliphatic aldehydes | 1.1% |
| | ketones | 3.6% |
| | sesquiterpenes | 29.1% |
| | lactones & coumarins | |
| | remainder | 8.5% |
| | oxides | 1.1% |
| | acids | trace |
| | aromatic aldehydes | trace |
| | monoterpenes | 23.6% |
| | alcohols | 29.8% |
| | phenols, phe. ethers | 1.6% |

**CCP of BLEND RECIPE**

*Patchouli* (pogostemon cablin)

*Myrrh* (commiphora myrrha)

*Cypress* (cupressus sempervirens)

*Patchouli* is antiviral, astringent, bactericidal, decongestant and a tonic to the immune system. It is recommended for phlebitis and varicose veins. It heals damaged tissue. The aroma is sweet and earthy.

*Myrrh* is antiinflammatory, antifungal, antiseptic and astringent. It is excellent for helping skin tissue repair.

*Cypress* is astringent, contracts the blood vessels and is a decongestant. It is recommended for broken capillaries, haemorrhoids, rheumatism and sweaty feet.

*Chemical constituents to be found in the blend may include:*

- myrrholic ester, α-terpinyl acetate
- 2-butanal
- patchoulenone, isopatchoulenone, methyl isobutyl ketone, curzerenone
- α-guaiene, patchoulenes, elemene, cedrene, cadinene, α-bulnesene, seychellenes, caryophyllene, copaene
- guaiene oxide, bulnesene oxide, caryophyllene oxide, 1.8-cineole

- myrrholic acid
- cinnamaldehyde, cuminaldehyde
- α-pinene, β-pinene, Δ3-carene, p-cymene, camphene, limonene, dipentene
- guaiol, bulnesol, pogostol, cedrol, patchouli alcohols, myrrh alcohols, α-terpineol, borneol, sabinol
- eugenol

## BLEND

| | |
|---|---|
| 6 drops | *Patchouli* |
| 27 drops | *Myrrh* |
| <u>15 drops</u> | *Cypress* |
| <u>48 drops</u> | *BLEND* |

Make up your *BLEND* using the quantities above – store in a small dark glass bottle fitted with a dropper.

## AILMENT

Haemorrhoids are distended veins in the rectum about one inch above the anus. Lack of dietary fibre leading to constipation may be the cause of them forming. Once the pain and discomfort of haemorrhoids is present that also sets up constipation so there is a vicious circle to break. Another cause of haemorrhoids is the pressure on the veins by a pregnant uterus. Thus haemorrhoids are a common occurrence during pregnancy. Any compression of the veins can cause haemorrhoids.

Fortunately although a nuisance, haemorrhoids usually heal up given careful attention. However it is advisable to get a medical diagnosis to confirm that the bleeding is due to haemorrhoids. The early stages of cancer have very similar symptoms so it's well worth checking up.

## BATHS

Add 8 drops of *BLEND* to your bath. Take frequent baths soaking and relaxing in them is very beneficial. If you have a sitz bath this is ideal.

## APPLICATION

Add 12 drops of *BLEND* to 30 ml of KY jelly. Rub this all around the anal area. Repeat this 2 or 3 times a day.

## LIFE STYLE

Take time to rest regularly to relieve the pressure on the veins. Always rest with your feet raised. In pregnancy take regular 10 minute rests throughout the day. This is very beneficial and will keep your energy levels up.

## SUPPOSITORIES

Chemists can supply you with suppositories which can be extremely helpful with the discomfort experienced with haemorrhoids.

## DIET

Try to avoid getting constipated. Follow a wholefood diet with a good level of fibre.

# Headaches

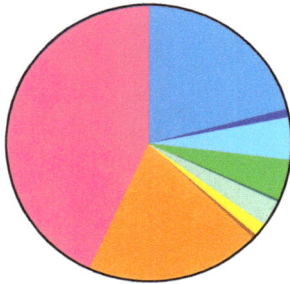

| | |
|---|---|
| esters | 21.6% |
| aliphatic aldehydes | 0.9% |
| ketones | 5.1% |
| sesquiterpenes | 4.2% |
| lactones & coumarins | 0.1% |
| remainder | 2.9% |
| oxides | 1.7% |
| acids | trace |
| aromatic aldehydes | 0.4% |
| monoterpenes | 20.2% |
| alcohols | 42.9% |
| phenols, phe. ethers | trace |

**CCP of BLEND RECIPE**

*Lavender True* (lavandula angustifolia)

*Marjoram Sweet* (origanum majorana)

*Mint Peppermint* (mentha piperita)

*Lavender True* is analgesic, antispasmodic, balancing and calming. It lowers blood pressure and is recommended for anxiety, headaches, insomnia and migraines.

*Marjoram Sweet*, known as 'joy of the mountain', is analgesic, antispasmodic, balancing and helps with depression and headaches. It is recommended for clearing obsessional thought patterns.

*Mint Peppermint* acts as a local anaesthetic and is helpful to mental fatigue, nervous exhaustion migraines and stress.

*Chemical constituents to be found in the blend may include:*

- linalyl acetate, terpinyl acetate, geranyl acetate, menthyl acetate, lavandulyl acetate
- citral
- menthone, isomenthone, pulegone, octanone, camphor
- germacrene, β-caryophyllene
- aesculetine, menthofuran, coumarin
- 1.8-cineole, caryophyllene oxide
- cuminaldehyde, benzaldehyde
- β-pinene, α-terpinene, γ-terpinene, p-cymene, myrcene, limonene, ocimene, sabinene, α-pinene
- terpinen-4-ol, α-terpineol, linalool, borneol, geraniol, lavandulol, menthol, neomenthol
- carvacrol, eugenol

## BLEND

20 drops   *Lavender True*
20 drops   *Marjoram Sweet*
 5 drops   *Mint Peppermint*
45 drops   *BLEND*

Make up your *BLEND* using the quantities above – store in a small dark glass bottle fitted with a dropper.

## AILMENT

Everybody experiences headaches. Unfortunately it is almost impossible to be sure of the causes. It can be part of any illness from a small boil to high blood pressure. The meninges that cover the brain are the tissues that perceive the pain as the brain itself is fairly insensitive. If something irritates the meninges this irritation is likely to manifest itself as a headache. For some chronic headache sufferers it proves very difficult to pinpoint the causes.

Migraine, the most extreme form of headaches, is equally difficult to tie down to a single cause. All that can be said is that a headache is triggered by the blood vessels in the head. An exception to this is sinusitis where the pain is related to the bone of the skull.

However despite the difficulty in tracking down the many causes of headaches by far the most common cause is over tiredness and anxiety. In these states the muscles of the neck and shoulders tense up and the pressure results in a headache.

Severe and sudden headpain or headaches that persist long term should be reported to your doctor to check that no serious condition is causing pressure to build up.

## MASSAGE

Make up a bottle of Headache Treatment Oil by adding 12 drops of *BLEND* to 30 ml of Sweet Almond Oil.

Headaches that start at the back of the head are almost certain to be caused by muscle tension. Get a friend to massage your neck. Gentle strokes down the back of the neck, firmer pressure around the shoulders and kneading action on the tight muscle band each side of the neck.

## TISSUES

Place 2 drops of *BLEND* on a tissue and inhale at frequent intervals. Pop prepared tissues in your pocket.

## BATHS

Add 8 drops of *BLEND* to your baths. Soak and relax.

## APPLICATION

Place 2 drops of *Lavender True* on your fingers and rub gently around your temples. Also rub your fingers across the back of your neck. Try to lie down away from the light and close your eyes for a rest period.

Pinching the bridge of your nose may also help.

Hot and cold compresses may also lessen the pain by stimulating the circulation.

## DIET

Avoid chocolate, cheese and red wine if you suffer from migraine.

# Herpes Simplex

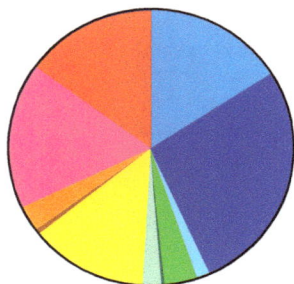

| | | |
|---|---|---|
| ■ | esters | 16.2% |
| ■ | aliphatic aldehydes | 27.0% |
| ■ | ketones | 1.5% |
| ■ | sesquiterpenes | 3.3% |
| ■ | lactones & coumarins | 0.1% |
| ■ | remainder | 2.7% |
| ■ | oxides | 13.8% |
| ■ | acids | trace |
| ■ | aromatic aldehydes | 0.3% |
| ■ | monoterpenes | 3.0% |
| ■ | alcohols | 17.0% |
| ■ | phenols, phe. ethers | 15.1% |

**CCP of BLEND RECIPE**

*Eucalyptus Blue Gum* (eucalyptus globulus)

*Eucalyptus Lemon Scented* (eucalyptus citriodora)

*Clove Bud* (syzygium aromaticum)

*Lavender True* (lavandula angustifolia)

*Eucalyptus Blue Gum* is antiseptic and decongestant. Recommended for chicken pox, herpes simplex and measles.

*Eucalyptus Lemon Scented* is antiviral, bactericidal and used to treat scabs, sores, herpes simplex and chicken pox.

*Clove Bud* is a powerful oil used to clear skin problems such as infected acne and herpes simplex blisters.

*Lavender True* excellent for helping damaged skin to heal.

*Chemical constituents to be found in the blend may include:*

- ■ linalyl acetate, geranyl acetate, lavandulyl acetate, citronellyl butyrate, α-terpinyl acetate citronellyl citronellate
- ■ citronellal, citral
- ■ menthone, pinocarvone, camphor
- ■ β-caryophyllene, humulenes, aromadendrene
- ■ coumarin, umbelliferone
- ■ 1.8-cineole, caryophyllene oxide
- ■ cuminaldehyde, benzaldehyde
- ■ α-pinene, limonene, *p*-cymene
- ■ citronellol, terpinen-4-ol, α-terpineol, borneol, linalool, lavandulol
- ■ eugenol, isoeugenol, aceteugenol

## BLEND

| | |
|---|---|
| 7 drops | *Eucalyptus Blue Gum* |
| 14 drops | *Eucalyptus Lemon Scented* |
| 7 drops | *Clove bud* |
| 14 drops | *Lavender True* |
| 42 drops | *BLEND* |

Make up your *BLEND* using the quantities above – store in a small dark glass bottle fitted with a dropper.

## AILMENT

Herpes simplex is a virus that once in the body lies dormant in a nerve ganglion. It can erupt at any time.

There are 2 different strains of this virus.

Herpes Simplex Type I is the well known cold sore. Almost everybody is infected with this virus having come into contact with it as a child. The eruptions can appear anywhere but most commonly they appear on the face near the mouth. The virus erupts when the body system is depleted due to some other infection. This is why cold sores so often appear during a cold. They are tiresome but harmless. However they can become dangerous if contracted by a baby prone to allergic eczema and also if they break out near the eyes. In either of these cases seek medical advice.

Herpes Simplex Type II causes similar lesions but it attacks the sexual organs and is called genital herpes. It is much more common now and is registered as a sexually transmitted disease. The initial attack of genital herpes is quite distressing. The sufferer will feel ill and the attack will take 10 days or so to run its course. Subsequent attacks are not so severe.

Herpes zoster is the chicken pox and shingles virus. In the case of shingles it is advisable to seek medical advice as once again it become very dangerous if it attacks the eyes.

There is no known cure for this virus.

## TREATMENT

Keep the lesions clean and dry. As the virus can be transferred to the eyes keep your fingers away from your eyes. Use clean flannels and towels every day.

## APPLICATION

Make up a bottle of Herpes Simplex Treatment Oil by adding 12 drops of *BLEND* to 30 ml of Sweet Almond Oil and 5 drops of Calendula Oil.

To ease the discomfort, gentle apply the Treatment Oil, using cotton wool pads, to the affected parts 2 or 3 times daily.

## BATHS

To ease the discomfort from genital herpes put 8 drops of *BLEND* in your bath. Soak and relax twice a day.

## DIET

Try to build up your immune system so that the body is not prone to attacks of the herpes virus.

**Daily Supplements**
Multi vitamin/mineral tablet
Vitamin C    1000 mgs

# Impetigo

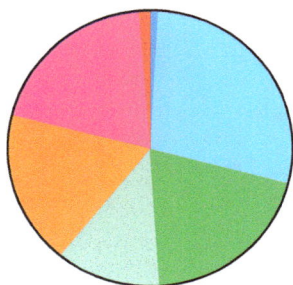

| | | |
|---|---|---|
| ■ | esters | trace |
| ■ | aliphatic aldehydes | 1.0% |
| ■ | ketones | 28.0% |
| ■ | sesquiterpenes | 19.5% |
| ■ | lactones & coumarins | trace |
| ■ | remainder | 12.5% |
| ■ | oxides | |
| ■ | acids | trace |
| ■ | aromatic aldehydes | trace |
| ■ | monoterpenes | 17.5% |
| ■ | alcohols | 20.0% |
| ■ | phenols, phe. ethers | 1.5% |

**CCP of BLEND RECIPE**

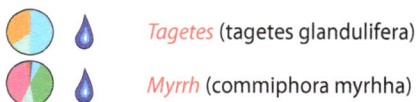

 🌢  *Tagetes* (tagetes glandulifera)

 🌢  *Myrrh* (commiphora myrhha)

*Tagetes* is antiseptic, antifungal, bactericidal, antiinflammatory and helps to generate new cell growth to repair damaged skin. It is recommended for many skin related problems such as corns, callouses, infected sores. The aroma is a strong pungent marigold – the plants are known to deter pests and are often planted to protect other plants from damage.

*Myrrh* is well known to help serious skin conditions such as ulcers, gangrene and bed sores. It is antiviral, antiseptic, antiinflammatory. The oil has a drying effect which helps healing to occur. The aroma is musky and smoky.

This blend produces a very earthy aroma.

---

*Chemical constituents to be found in the blend may include:*

- ■ myrrholic ester
- ■ citral, 2-butanal
- ■ tagetone, tagetenones, carvone, methyl isobutyl ketone, curzerenone
- ■ elemene, heerabolene, cadinene, copaene, curzerene, lindestrene
- ■ myrrholic acid
- ■ cinnamaldehyde, cuminaldehyde, salicylaldehyde
- ■ pinenes, limonene, ocimene, myrcene, camphene, limonene
- ■ linalool, myrrh alcohols
- ■ eugenol

## BLEND

16 drops   *Tagetes*
<u>16 drops</u>   *Myrrh*
<u>32 drops</u>   *BLEND*

Make up your *BLEND* using the quantities above – store in a small dark glass bottle fitted with a dropper.

## AILMENT

Impetigo is a highly contagious bacterial infection of the skin. Outbreaks at schools occur from time to time and if not checked quickly a minor epidemic can occur. The sores are particularly unsightly and will persist for a long time if not treated properly. Although a child will not feel ill they remain highly infectious. The staphylococci actually form small clusters of abscesses which show up as red spots with yellow crusts. They usually affect sufferer's face, hands or knees.

## TREATMENT

As soon as the condition is recognised it is important to start careful treatment. If not attended to the infection will spread to other parts of the skin making the healing process more difficult.

First of all attend to the infected pus to keep the area as clean as possible. Prepare a bowl of cool boiled water and add 5 drops of *Lavender True* (lavandula angustifolia). Using cotton wool pads gentle wash the pus from the sores. Use fresh cotton wool each time so that the water remains clean from infection.

With a fresh bowl of water again with 5 drops of *Lavender True* prepare a compress using a clean cotton cloth. Soak the cloth in the water and then gently lay it on the sores. Hold in place for a few minutes.

## COMPRESSES

For a compress that will be left in place prepare a large bowl of just boiled water. Cut a piece of lint that is double the size of the area you wish to treat. Put 2 drops of *BLEND* in the water and soak the lint then wring it out. Fold the lint in half and place in position. Either bandage it or if necessary use plaster tape to secure it.

Leave the lint in position for 2 to 3 hours then leave the sore open to the air.

It will take time and patience to encourage the sores to heal but essential oils are exceptionally helpful.

Make sure that the sufferer is unlikely to pass the infection on. If necessary, they should stay at home for a few days.

## BATHS

Put 4 drops of *BLEND* in baths.

# Indigestion

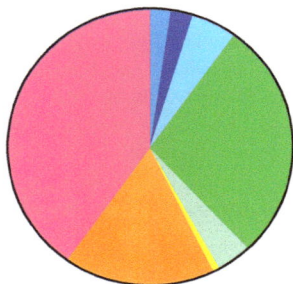

| | | |
|---|---|---|
| ■ | esters | 2.5% |
| ■ | aliphatic aldehydes | 2.5% |
| ■ | ketones | 5.0% |
| ■ | sesquiterpenes | 27.5% |
| ■ | lactones & coumarins | trace |
| ■ | remainder | 4.3% |
| ■ | oxides | 0.7% |
| ■ | acids | trace |
| ■ | aromatic aldehydes | |
| ■ | monoterpenes | 17.5% |
| ■ | alcohols | 40.0% |
| ■ | phenols, phe. ethers | trace |

**CCP of BLEND RECIPE**

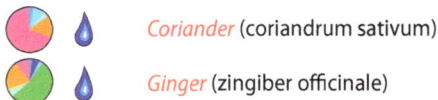

*Coriander* (coriandrum sativum)

*Ginger* (zingiber officinale)

*Coriander* has a sweet spicy woody aroma. It has been used since ancient times – considered the herb of happiness. It is a tonic to the digestive system and helps with colic, bad breath, anorexia, enteritis and indigestion. It belongs to the Umbelliferae botanical family which is known to aid digestion.

*Ginger* has a warm pleasant spicy aroma and is a very comforting oil. It is useful for helping hangovers, indigestion, flatulence, nausea and seasickness. It is an analgesic, antispasmodic and prevents stomach griping. It is used in many ancient remedies. The oil is distilled from unpeeled dried ground rhizome.

---

*Chemical constituents to be found in the blend may include:*

- ■ geranyl acetate, linalyl acetate
- ■ decyl aldehyde, geranial, citronellal
- ■ camphor, carvone, gingerone
- ■ β-sesquiphellandrene, zingiberene, *ar*-curcumene
- ■ umbelliferone, bergaptene

- ■ 1.8-cineole
- ■ γ-terpinene, *p*-cymene, α-pinene, limonene, β-pinene, camphene
- ■ linalool, α-terpineol, geraniol, citronellol, borneol, gingerol
- ■ anethole

## BLEND

20 drops   *Coriander*
20 drops   *Ginger*
40 drops   *BLEND*

Make up your *BLEND* using the quantities above – store in a small dark glass bottle fitted with a dropper.

## AILMENT

For indigestion due to flatulence consult the notes on Gastric Flatulence.

Indigestion may take the form of the regurgitation of acid, or partly digested food, from the stomach into the oesophagus. This results in the pain commonly described as heart burn and another term to describe the indigestion is 'acid stomach'.

This reaction from the stomach can be caused by overeating, constricted clothing, obesity and physical exercise immediately after eating.

However regular attacks can also be caused by a loose muscle in the oesophagus that allows the acid back from the stomach. A more serious cause of the acid could be a stomach ulcer. If you suffer continuously from poor digestion seek medical advice.

## COMPRESSES

Prepare a bowl of hot water and place 4 drops of *BLEND* in it. Using a cotton cloth make a warm compress by soaking the cloth in the prepared water. Wring out and place across the top of the abdomen where the discomfort is experienced.

## MASSAGE

Make up a bottle of Indigestion Treatment Oil by adding 12 drops of *BLEND* to 30 ml of Sweet Almond Oil.

Massage the Treatment Oil gently around the top of the abdomen. Do this between meals to help to calm the system down. Use gentle circular movements.

## TISSUES

Put a 3 drops of *BLEND* onto a tissue. Inhale whenever the pain occurs. Take deep slow breathes.

## LIFE STYLE

Spend 20 minutes winding down before eating and 20 minutes to allow digestion of the food after eating. This can make a great difference to the amount of discomfort you experience. Also eat slowly and deliberately chewing all your food thoroughly as this is the first part of the digestive action and one that you can control. Don't smoke – this irritates the stomach lining.

Try to reduce your stress level to a minimum.

## DIET

Cut out fatty foods and those that contain food additives and spices. Eat small and regular meals.

Avoid aspirin as it harms the stomach lining.

# Leg Ulcers

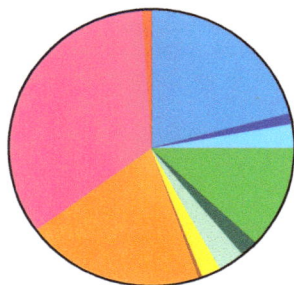

| | | |
|---|---|---|
| | esters | 21.2% |
| | aliphatic aldehydes | 1.0% |
| | ketones | 2.5% |
| | sesquiterpenes | 12.6% |
| | lactones & coumarins | 1.3% |
| | remainder | 3.8% |
| | oxides | 2.3% |
| | acids | trace |
| | aromatic aldehydes | 0.3% |
| | monoterpenes | 19.5% |
| | alcohols | 34.7% |
| | phenols, phe. ethers | 0.8% |

**CCP of BLEND RECIPE**

*Lavender True* (lavandula angustifolia)

*Tea Tree* (melaleuca alternifolia)

*Bergamot* (citrus bergamia)

*Myrrh* (commiphora myrrha)

*Lavender True* is excellent for the regeneration of skin cells. It heals wounds and scars and is on the whole a calming oil.

*Tea Tree* is strongly antiseptic which helps to protect the wound from infection.

*Bergamot* calms anxiety. It also assists skin to heal. It can be most helpful at combating depression.

*Myrrh* has a good drying effect on the skin. It will help the skin heal and also is calming to the nervous system.

All the chemical families are present in this blend with the esters, sesquiterpenes, monoterpenes and alcohols being the largest proportions.

*Chemical constituents to be found in the blend may include:*

- linalyl acetate, lavandulyl acetate
- cadinene, β-caryophyllene, elemene
- α-pinene, β-pinene, γ-terpinene, α-terpinene, *p*-cymene
- α-terpineol, linalool, geraniol, myrrh alcohols, terpinen-4-ol, borneol, lavandulol

## BLEND

| 10 drops | *Lavender True* |
|---|---|
| 10 drops | *Tea Tree* |
| 10 drops | *Bergamot* |
| <u>10 drops</u> | *Myrrh* |
| <u>40 drops</u> | *BLEND* |

Make up your *BLEND* using the quantities above – store in a small dark glass bottle fitted with a dropper.

## WATER SPRAY

Put 2 drops of the *BLEND* into a small cup of warm water. Put this into a fine water sprayer. If possible keep the wound open to the air and spray the ulcer regularly. When it is necessary to cover the ulcer for protection or for sleeping take a melamine dressing and before laying it over the ulcer spray it with the Treatment Water.

Make up a fresh cup of Treatment Water each day.

Persevere with this treatment keeping the ulcer open to the air when possible.

It may sting a little when you spray the ulcer.

Ulcers are very persistent, treatment will take 1-2 months to work.

Take great care of the wound area.

## BATHS

If your doctor allows you to bath then add 8 drops of the *BLEND* to your bath water. This will keep the wound antiseptic.

## COMPRESSES

Add 12 drops of the *BLEND* to 30 ml of calendula oil. Gently massage a little of this Treatment Oil into the leg surrounding the wound. Allow a little of it to run onto the wound but do not actually touch the wound. Cut a soft cotton sheet to form a wadding to lay over the wound. Prepare some Treatment Water by putting 8 drops of *BLEND* into a basin of warm water.

Soak the wadding in the treatment water. Squeeze out the wadding and lay it gently over the wound. Wrap cling film around the leg to hold the compress in place. Wrap a towel round to keep the warmth in. Leave in place for at least half an hour and longer if possible. The warmth encourages the circulation and helps the oils to penetrate the skin.

## DRINK

Put one teaspoon of honey into a cup of hot water, add 1 drop of *Mint Peppermint* (mentha piperita).

Sip this drink slowly concentrating on relaxing. Rest with your feet raised.

## FOOT MASSAGE

To help the circulation a daily foot massage is highly recommended. If possible book a treatment with a qualified reflexologist.

## DIET

Take Zinc, Vitamins E, C, D, also beta-carotene (A) and garlic tablets. Cook with plenty of garlic and onions.

Reduce intake of dairy products Drink herbal teas. Eat raw parsley.

# Measles

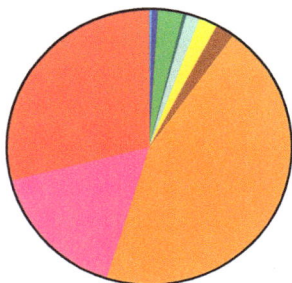

| | | |
|---|---|---|
| | esters | 0.2% |
| | aliphatic aldehydes | 0.5% |
| | ketones | trace |
| | sesquiterpenes | 3.3% |
| | lactones & coumarins | 0.2% |
| | remainder | 1.5% |
| | oxides | 2.3% |
| | acids | trace |
| | aromatic aldehydes | 1.7% |
| | monoterpenes | 45.7% |
| | alcohols | 16.0% |
| | phenols, phe. ethers | 28.6% |

**CCP of BLEND RECIPE**

 *Cinnamon Leaf* (cinnamomum zeylanicum)

 *Grapefruit* (citrus paradisi)

 *Tea Tree* (melaleuca alternifolia)

*Cinnamon Leaf* is antiviral, bactericidal, antioxidant, and a stimulant. It acts as a blood purifier. It is a powerful oil and is always used with care – avoid in pregnancy. The aroma is musty sweet and sharp.

*Grapefruit* has a sharp refreshing aroma. It is a very steadying oil and can be used to alleviate stress headaches and migraine attacks. It is excellent for local infections and congested skin.

*Tea Tree* is antiviral and strongly bactericidal. It is an immune system tonic and stimulates the body's healing processes. Extensively used in aboriginal medicine – excellent for treating infected wounds.

*Chemical constituents to be found in the blend may include:*

- benzyl benzoate, benzyl acetate, cinnamyl acetate, geranyl acetate
- citronellal, citral, sinensal
- β-caryophyllene, cadinene, aromadendrene, viridiflorene
- auraptene, limettin
- 1.8-cineole, 1.4-cineole
- cinnamaldehyde, methyl vanillin
- α-pinene, α-terpinene, γ-terpinene, p-cymene, limonene, terpinolene
- terpinen-4-ol, α-terpineol, globulol, geraniol, linalool, paradisiol, borneol
- eugenol, safrole, aceteugenol

## BLEND

10 drops   *Cinnamon Leaf*
10 drops   *Grapefruit*
10 drops   *Tea Tree*
30 drops   *BLEND*

Make up your *BLEND* using the quantities above – store in a small dark glass bottle fitted with a dropper.

## AILMENT

Measles is a very common and contagious disease. The virus is transferred by airborne droplets and saliva. The incubation period is 7 to 14 days and the first symptoms to appear are a running nose and eyes followed by a sore throat and fever. Small red spots with white centres appear on the inside of the mouth – these are known as Kopliks spots. On the 4th day the blotchy skin rash spreads down the body starting from the face. The virus will run its course over the next 7 to 14 days. The dangerous aspect of measles is the fear of secondary infections. The body is particularly vulnerable to such complications as bronchitis, pneumonia, and ear infections that can lead to deafness.

It is necessary to take every precaution to prevent the sufferer becoming infected by other illnesses.

## ROOM SPRAY

Add 5 drops of *BLEND* per litre of water and fill up a plant spray. Spray all the rooms in the house, including the sick room. This is a precaution to keep secondary infections at bay.

## BODY LOTION

Make up a bottle of Measles Treatment Lotion by adding 5 drops of *Chamomile Roman* and 5 drops of *Lavender True* to 100 ml of Calamine Lotion.

Shake the bottle well and apply gently all over the rash to ease the discomfort.

## BATHS

Put 4 drops of *Chamomile Roman* in the bath.

## TREATMENT

Keep the sufferer in bed for a few days and isolated from others as far as possible. It can help to keep the room slightly darkened as the eyes can be sensitive to light.

Measles is mainly a childhood disease and an attack builds up immunity. A vaccine was introduced in the 1960s which has reduced the reported cases of the disease considerably. Adult sufferers are likely to feel quite ill and need to take care from contracting any secondary infections.

## DIET

Take Vitamin C 1000 mgs per day.

Stick to a light, easy to digest, diet.

Drink 8 glasses of mineral water a day.

# Menopause

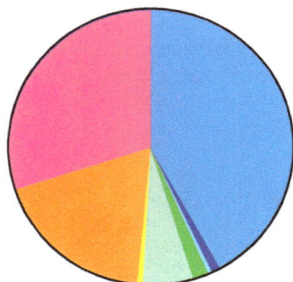

| | | |
|---|---|---|
| 🟦 | esters | 42.0% |
| 🟦 | aliphatic aldehydes | 1.0% |
| 🟦 | ketones | 0.3% |
| 🟩 | sesquiterpenes | 2.0% |
| 🟩 | lactones & coumarins | trace |
| 🟩 | remainder | 5.8% |
| 🟨 | oxides | 0.4% |
| 🟨 | acids | trace |
| 🟫 | aromatic aldehydes | |
| 🟧 | monoterpenes | 18.5% |
| 🟥 | alcohols | 30.0% |
| 🟧 | phenols, phe. ethers | trace |

**CCP of BLEND RECIPE**

*Orange Blossom Neroli* (citrus aurantium amara)

*Clary Sage* (salvia sclarea)

*Orange Blossom Neroli* is analgesic, aphrodisiac and antiaging. The aroma is haunting and beautiful. The oil is very powerful for emotional problems. It has a balancing effect and is recommended for both menopausal problems and pre-menstrual tension.

*Clary Sage* is often called a woman's oil because of its oestrogen like action. It is calming, sedative and lowers blood pressure. The aroma is nutty and earthy. It is particularly recommended for menopausal problems.

Because of its hormone-like action avoid in cases of hormone related cancers. Also avoid in pregnancy and do not use if alcohol has been consumed.

*Chemical constituents to be found in the blend may include:*

🟦 methyl anthranilate, linalyl acetate, geranyl acetate, neryl acetate
🟦 caryophyllenal
🟦 jasmone, thujone, camphor
🟩 caryophyllene, germacrene, bourbonene
🟩 indole

🟨 1.8-cineole, caryophyllene oxide
🟨 phenylacetic acid
🟧 α-pinene, β-pinene, myrcene, limonene, phellandrene
🟥 linalool, sclareol, α-terpineol, nerol, α-bisabolol, geraniol, nerolidol, benzyl alcohol, phenylethyl alcohol
🟧 methyl hexyl ether

## BLEND

20 drops *Orange Blossom Neroli*
20 drops *Clary Sage*
40 drops *BLEND*

Make up your *BLEND* using the quantities above – store in a small dark glass bottle fitted with a dropper.

## AILMENT

The menopause is not an ailment as such – it is just a natural ageing process. The ovaries cease to release an egg cell each month as the pituitary gland's and ovary's hormones change. The normal age for the menopause falls between 40 and 50 years old but there are many exceptions to this. Some women suffer extremely early onset of the menopause.

For many women the 'change of life' as it is called causes no problems whatsoever. For others the change proves quite distressing.

Actual physical phenomenon are the occurrence of 'hot flushes'. Not everybody experiences these and they normally cease after a few months and are mainly just an irritating discomfort. The more serious physical change in the body is the gradual loss of density from the bones that can lead to osteoporosis in later years. If there is a family history of bad osteoporosis it may be advisable to take Hormone Replacement Therapy (HRT) for a few years. Take medical advice on this. The emotional reaction to the hormonal change in the body is more complicated to deal with. Some women suffer depression which may be due not so much to the change of hormones as to the change of life style. Such things as all the children leaving home, new career patterns and so on all occur at this time.

## MASSAGE

Make up a bottle of Menopause Treatment Oil by adding 12 drops of *BLEND* to 30 ml of Sweet Almond Oil.

Get a friend to give you a full body massage with this Treatment Oil at least once a week. Better still treat yourself to a regular visit to an aromatherapist. Taking time out for yourself will help tremendously with feelings of depression that can occur as you adjust to new life styles. The oils will work gently to restore a hormonal balance and the aromatherapist's experience and advice will help you understand why you are experiencing problems.

## BATHS

Put 8 drops of *BLEND* in your bath. Soak and relax.

## LIFE STYLE

Major desire at this time is to feel 'needed'. Work on positive ways of achieving this with new activities.

## TISSUES

Put 1 drop of *Mint Peppermint* on a tissue. Inhale during 'hot flushes'.

## DIET

Muti-vitamin tablets. Drink plenty of mineral water.

# Mumps

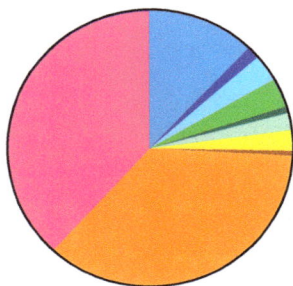

| | | |
|---|---|---|
| | esters | 12.3% |
| | aliphatic aldehydes | 1.0% |
| | ketones | 3.0% |
| | sesquiterpenes | 3.3% |
| | lactones & coumarins | 0.6% |
| | remainder | 2.2% |
| | oxides | 2.3% |
| | acids | trace |
| | aromatic aldehydes | 0.3% |
| | monoterpenes | 36.8% |
| | alcohols | 38.2% |
| | phenols, phe. ethers | trace |

**CCP of BLEND RECIPE**

 🌢 *Tea Tree* (melaleuca alternifolia)

 🌢 *Lavender True* (lavandula angustifolia)

 🌢 *Coriander* (coriandrum sativum)

 🌢 *Lemon* (citrus limon)

*Tea Tree* is antiviral, strongly bactericidal, decongestant and an immune system stimulant.

*Lavender True* is antiviral, analgesic, calming and balancing. It will help alleviate headaches and discomfort.

*Coriander* is analgesic and antiviral. It has a comforting sweet spicy woody aroma which blends well with the other oils.

*Lemon* is a decongestant and cleanses the body systems.

*Chemical constituents to be found in the blend may include:*

- linalyl acetate, geranyl acetate, neryl acetate, terpinyl acetate
- citral, citronellal, nonanal, octanal
- octanone, camphor, carvone
- β-bisabolene, α-bergamotene, aromadendrene, viridiflorene
- bergaptene, bergamottin, coumarin, umbelliferone
- 1.8-cineole, linalool oxide
- cuminaldehyde, benzaldehyde
- α-pinene, α-terpinene, γ-terpinene, terpinolene, p-cymene, myrcene, limonene, sabinene
- terpinen-4-ol, α-terpineol, linalool, borneol, geraniol, lavandulol
- anethole

## BLEND

| 10 drops | *Tea Tree* |
| 10 drops | *Lavender True* |
| 10 drops | *Coriander* |
| 10 drops | *Lemon* |
| 40 drops | *BLEND* |

Make up your *BLEND* using the quantities above – store in a small dark glass bottle fitted with a dropper.

## AILMENT

Mumps is a common virus disease that most people get during childhood. The virus is similar to an influenza virus and is airborne. The first signs of mumps appear 2 to 4 weeks after exposure to the virus. It starts with a mild temperature and then the parotid salivary glands swell up painfully. This shows as an egg shaped swelling in front of the ear over the angle of the jaw bone.

Sometimes the face just swells on the one side. The swelling usually subsides after a day or two.

Occasionally the virus attacks other salivary glands and less often the testes or pancreas. As with most virus infections the nervous system may become involved. Earache often accompanies mumps and is particularly painful when eating.

Normally the symptoms are mild and short lived.

If contracted as an adult, it can cause sterility in men and there have been cases where diabetes was triggered. However these are rare occurrences.

## ROOM SPRAY

Add 5 drops of *BLEND* per pint of water and fill up a plant spray. Spray rooms in the house and especially in the sick room.

## APPLICATION

Make up a bottle of Mumps Treatment Oil by adding 12 drops of *BLEND* to 30 ml of Sweet Almond Oil.

Apply the treatment oil gently and carefully to the sore area. Also apply to the back of the neck and the abdominal area. Repeat the application 3 times daily.

## TREATMENT

A few days rest are advisable to give the body support to deal with the virus. It will take its course. The oils will help with the pain and discomfort. Take mild pain killers if necessary.

## DIET

The dryness in the mouth can be helped with a mouth wash.

Easy to eat foods are a good idea because of the pain in the jaw.

Soups and easy to digest foods. Avoid any acid drinks such as orange juice.

Take supplements to boost the immune system.

Drink plenty of spring water.

# Osteoarthritis

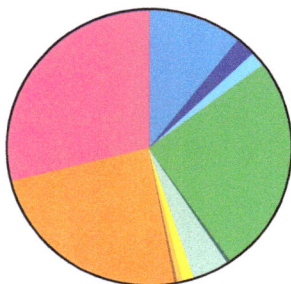

| | | |
|---|---|---|
| ■ | esters | 10.8% |
| ■ | aliphatic aldehydes | 2.2% |
| ■ | ketones | 1.6% |
| ■ | sesquiterpenes | 25.6% |
| ■ | lactones & coumarins | 0.1% |
| ■ | remainder | 4.9% |
| ■ | oxides | 1.1% |
| ■ | acids | 0.5% |
| ■ | aromatic aldehydes | 0.2% |
| ■ | monoterpenes | 23.8% |
| ■ | alcohols | 29.2% |
| ■ | phenols, phe. ethers | trace |

**CCP of BLEND RECIPE**

*Lavender True* (lavandula angustifolia)

*Cypress* (cupressus sempervirens)

*Sandalwood* (santalum album)

*Ginger* (zingiber officinale)

*Lavender True* is an antiinflammatory and an analgesic. It is a soothing and balancing oil.
*Cypress* balances the sympathetic nerve system. It is a decongestant and recommended for rheumatism.
*Sandalwood* is an antiinflammatory and helpful for lumbago.
*Ginger* is an analgesic, good for arthritis and back pains – a warming oil.

*Chemical constituents to be found in the blend may include:*

■ linalyl acetate, lavandulyl acetate, α-terpinyl acetate, terpinen-4-yl acetate

■ citral, geranial, citronellal

■ octanone, camphor, santalone, gingerone

■ β-caryophyllene, cedrene, santalenes, β-sesquiphellandrene, zingiberene

■ coumarin, umbelliferone

■ 1.8-cineole, manoyl oxide, linalool oxide, caryophyllene oxide

■ nortricycloekasantalic acid

■ cuminaldehyde, benzaldehyde

■ camphene, limonene, α-pinene, β-pinene, Δ3-carene, *p*-cymene

■ terpinen-4-ol, α-terpineol, linalool, borneol, geraniol, lavandulol sabinol, cedrol, santalols, gingerol

## BLEND

| 8 drops | *Lavender True* |
| 8 drops | *Cypress* |
| 8 drops | *Sandalwood* |
| <u>16 drops</u> | *Ginger* |
| <u>40 drops</u> | *BLEND* |

Make up your *BLEND* using the quantities above – store in a small dark glass bottle fitted with a dropper.

## AILMENT

Osteoarthritis is the degeneration of joints with some loss of the almost frictionless cartilage lining and the formation of rough deposits of bone. It is an inevitable aging process but can occur in middle age if joints have been subjected to abnormal use or pressure. Such pressure can be caused by something as simple as poor posture, injury or athletic activities can trigger the condition.

At first there are no symptoms of the cartilage loss but it first shows up as discomfort, pain and loss of movement.

If the pain becomes chronic and severe sometimes the only way to get relief from it is to undergo surgery.

The Hip Replacement operation has brought relief to countless sufferers giving them back a quality of life free of pain and with mobility restored.

Some operations 'fix' the painful joint. In this case the mobility is lost but the pain also vanishes.

## BATHS

Put 8 drops of *BLEND* in your bath. Soak and relax. This will help the pain.

## MASSAGE

Make up a bottle of Osteoarthritis Treatment Oil by adding 12 drops of *BLEND* to 30 ml of Sweet Almond Oil.

Massage the Treatment Oil gently around the affected joints. With osteoarthritis the connective tissue around the joint thickens and fluid may fill the joint. The essential oils will help to disperse this fluid.

Repeat the massage 2 or 3 times daily.

## TREATMENT

The degeneration of the joint cartilage can start quite innocently the only symptoms being an occasional ache and stiffness.

However a more ominous 'creaking' sound when the joint is moved heralds the onset of more breakdown of movement. One thing that is essential is to make sure that you keep the joint moving every day otherwise immobility can set in.

If a joint is particularly painful make up a small 30 ml pot of cream and add 12 drops of *Mint Peppermint* to it. Apply the ointment around the painful joint the *Mint Peppermint* will act as a local anaesthetic for a while.

## DIET

Drink plenty of mineral water. Cod liver oil capsules daily. Fresh fruits and vegetables.

It is worth consulting a diet expert and having a personal food plan built up.

# Periods – heavy

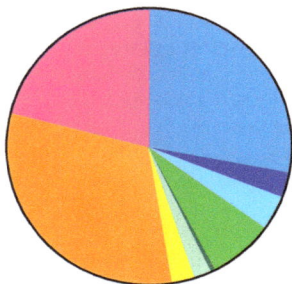

| | |
|---|---|
| esters | 27.6% |
| aliphatic aldehydes | 3.0% |
| ketones | 3.9% |
| sesquiterpenes | 7.3% |
| lactones & coumarins | 0.6% |
| remainder | 2.0% |
| oxides | 2.8% |
| acids | trace |
| aromatic aldehydes | |
| monoterpenes | 31.0% |
| alcohols | 21.8% |
| phenols, phe. ethers | trace |

**CCP of BLEND RECIPE**

*Yarrow* (achillea millefolium)

*Chamomile Roman* (chamaemelum nobile)

*Geranium* (pelargonium graveolens)

*Lemon* (citrus limon)

*Yarrow* is antispasmodic and decongestant. A good women's oil. It should be avoided in pregnancy.

*Chamomile Roman* is antispasmodic, calming and soothing.

*Geranium* is analgesic, helps with anxiety and generally balances the body.

*Lemon* is antispasmodic, calming and clarifying. It lowers blood pressure and generally cleanses the body.

*Chemical constituents to be found in the blend may include:*

- bornyl acetate, angelates, tiglates, neryl acetate, citronellyl formate
- citral, citronellal, nonanal
- isoartemisia, camphor, pinocarvone, menthone, thujone
- chamazulene, caryophyllene, germacrene, dihydroazulene, β-bisabolene, α-bergamotene
- achilline, bergaptene, bergamottin
- 1.8-cineole, *cis*-rose oxide
- imonene, α-pinene, β-pinene, γ-terpinene, *p*-cymene, sabinene, myrcene, camphene
- citronellol, geraniol, linalool
- eugenol

## BLEND

| 4 drops | *Yarrow* |
| 12 drops | *Chamomile Roman* |
| 12 drops | *Geranium* |
| 12 drops | *Lemon* |
| 40 drops | *BLEND* |

Make up your *BLEND* using the quantities above – store in a small dark glass bottle fitted with a dropper.

## AILMENT

Heavy bleeding during the monthly menstruation, or clotting in the normal flow or irregular bleeding at any time of the month is known as menorrhagia.

If you are a chronic sufferer of any of these conditions you need to seek advice to track down the causes.

Uterine bleeding can be a sign of uterine cancer or of a fibrous growth in the womb. It is a simple minor operation for the hospital to check your womb and give a clear diagnostic report.

The occasional occurrence of the conditions is often due to a stressful life style and slight hormonal imbalance.

## TREATMENT

Make up a bottle of Heavy Periods Treatment Oil by adding 12 drops of *BLEND* to 30 ml of Sweet Almond Oil.

Take time out daily to massage your abdomen and lower back with the Treatment Oil.

Also organise to rest for 30 minutes in the middle of the day with your feet raised.

## LIFE STYLE

Make a plan of a regular routine for the whole month. Time table the massage sessions and rest sessions. It is not so much the length of time for each session that is so important as the regularity of them. The body needs to establish a peaceful rhythm in order to function effectively.

Join a yoga or meditation class and learn the art of relaxation.

Treat yourself to a monthly appointment with a qualified aromatherapist or reflexologist. They will help you establish a plan.

## BATHS

Put 8 drops of *BLEND* in your bath. Soak and relax.

## VAPOURISER

Put 4 drops of *BLEND* in a vapouriser in any room that you are working in. The molecules of oil will circulate and have a calming effect.

## DIET

Eat plenty of green leafy vegetables for their iron content.

### Daily Supplements
Multi-vitamin/mineral tablet
Vitamin B6    100 mgs
Vitamin C    1000 mgs
Oil of Evening Primrose as per container.

# Periods – lack of

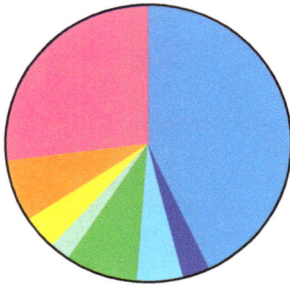

| | | |
|---|---|---|
| | esters | 43.4% |
| | aliphatic aldehydes | 2.9% |
| | ketones | 5.3% |
| | sesquiterpenes | 8.6% |
| | lactones & coumarins | trace |
| | remainder | 2.0% |
| | oxides | 4.1% |
| | acids | trace |
| | aromatic aldehydes | |
| | monoterpenes | 6.7% |
| | alcohols | 27.0% |
| | phenols, phe. ethers | trace |

## CCP of BLEND RECIPE

 *Yarrow* (achillea millefolium)

 *Chamomile Roman* (chamaemelum nobile)

 *Geranium* (pelargonium graveolens)

*Yarrow* is hormone like, stimulates secretions and is a good women's oil. Do not use during pregnancy. It is recommended for fibroids, ovaries, period problems and prolapse.

*Chamomile Roman* is a gentle calming oil. It will help anxiety and soothes the system. It is recommended for helping with the lack of periods (amenorrhoea) and nervous menstrual problems.

*Geranium* regulates hormone functions and generally balances the body. It helps with breast congestion, candida, painful periods, pmt and uterine haemorrhage.

### *Chemical constituents to be found in the blend may include:*

- bornyl acetate, citronellyl formate, angelates, tiglates, butyrates
- citral
- isoartemisia, camphor, thujone, pinocarvone, menthone
- chamazulene, caryophyllene, germacrene, dihydroazulene
- achilline
- 1.8-cineole, *cis*-rose oxide
- limonene, α-pinene, β-pinene, sabinene, camphene, myrcene
- citronellol, geraniol, linalool, farnesol, nerolidol, α-terpineol
- eugenol

## BLEND

| 5 drops | *Yarrow* |
|---|---|
| 20 drops | *Chamomile Roman* |
| <u>15 drops</u> | *Geranium* |
| <u>40 drops</u> | *BLEND* |

Make up your *BLEND* using the quantities above – store in a small dark glass bottle fitted with a dropper.

## AILMENT

The condition of the menstrual cycle stopping is called amenorrhoea. The menstrual cycle may cease due to a range of causes. A common cause is an emotional upset or even a physical shock. More serious causes include disease of the ovaries, some disturbance of the pituitary gland and anorexia.

One of the problems with restoring the cycle is that anxiety about a lack of periods is in itself an emotional upset. As with so many of the hormonal balances within the body it is necessary to remove as much stress from daily life as possible in order to give the body a chance to establish its correct rhythm.

During pregnancy it is natural that the menstrual cycle ceases. This is medically called secondary amenorrhoea and should not be confused the condition being discussed here which to be precise is called primary amenorrhoea.

The menstrual cycle usually starts from the age of 13 years onwards although for some girls it is earlier. However for some girls it starts much later. A lack of periods will often right itself when the sufferer's quality of life improves and/or their general health improves.

## TREATMENT

The best advice is to try keep your anxiety about the condition to a minimum. If you are feeling well in yourself the chances are that the body will restore its own rhythm. Essential oils are very helpful in balancing the endocrine system.

## MASSAGE

Make up a bottle of Lack of Periods Treatment Oil by adding 12 drops of *BLEND* to 30 ml of Sweet Almond Oil.

Massage the abdomen and lower back with the Treatment Oil 3 or 4 times a week.

Book a monthly appointment with an aromatherapist who will be able to help you with the anxiety that you may be feeling.

## BATHS

Put 8 drops of *BLEND* in your bath. Take your daily bath before going to bed. The oils will help to give you a peaceful sleep.

## LIFE STYLE

Consider how you can reduce stress in your life. Yoga classes may help.

## DIET

**Daily Supplements**
Multi-vitamin/mineral tablet
Vitamin B6    100 mgs
Vitamin C    1000 mgs

# Periods – painful

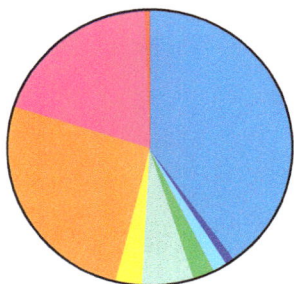

| | | |
|---|---|---|
| | esters | 39.8% |
| | aliphatic aldehydes | 1.1% |
| | ketones | 1.5% |
| | sesquiterpenes | 2.5% |
| | lactones & coumarins | trace |
| | remainder | 5.7% |
| | oxides | 2.8% |
| | acids | trace |
| | aromatic aldehydes | |
| | monoterpenes | 26.3% |
| | alcohols | 20.0% |
| | phenols, phe. ethers | 0.3% |

**CCP of BLEND RECIPE**

*Rose Otto* (rosa damascena)

*Cypress* (cupressus sempervirens)

*Chamomile Roman* (chamaemelum nobile)

*Rose Otto* is hormone like it regulates and stimulates the pituitary gland. It is antispasmodic, balancing and calming. The aroma is sweet, heavenly and flowery. It is a woman's oil that calms, relieves tension and feelings of inadequacy.

*Cypress* regulates the ovarian function and balances the sympathetic nerve system. It is recommended for irregular periods, menopause and pmt. The aroma is clear, woody and spicy.

*Chamomile Roman* is highly respected for its calming influence on all systems. It balances the menstrual cycle and helps with anaemia. The aroma is earthy, fruity and apple like.

*Chemical constituents to be found in the blend may include:*

- angelates, α-terpinyl acetate, tiglates, citronellyl acetate, geranyl acetate
- neral
- pinocarvone
- chamazulene, caryophyllene, cedrene, cadinene
- damascenone
- 1.8-cineole, manoyl oxide, rose oxide
- α-pinene, β-pinene, Δ3-carene, *p*-cymene, camphene, limonene, stearoptene, camphene, ocimene
- citronellol, geraniol, nerol, sabinol, α-terpineol, *trans*-pinocarveol
- methyl eugenol

## BLEND

10 drops   *Rose Otto*
10 drops   *Cypress*
<u>20 drops</u>   *Chamomile Roman*
<u>40 drops</u>   *BLEND*

Make up your *BLEND* using the quantities above – store in a small dark glass bottle fitted with a dropper.

## AILMENT

Many women are affected by menstrual pain just before and during their period.

The uterine cramps and sets up lower back and abdomen pains sometimes so severe that it is necessary to lie down until they ease up.

The whole episode can be made much worse if the situation is very stressful and there is no opportunity for relaxing and dealing with it.

If the severe pains are experienced every month for several days, it is wise to seek medical advice just in case it is a symptom of a more serious problem.

## TREATMENT

The best way to try and tackle this problem is to take some preventative measures.

The daily massage treatment described below should commence 14 days before your period is due. Keep your diary as clear as possible over the dates of your period. This will lift the level of anxiety that you may feel as the dates approach. Fear of pain can actually trigger a pain reaction.

## MASSAGE

Make up a bottle of Painful Periods Treatment Oil by adding 12 drops of *BLEND* to 30 ml of Sweet Almond Oil.

Apply the Treatment Oil each night to the small of the back and the lower abdomen. Gently massage over the abdomen with circular clock-wise strokes.

## BATHS

Put 8 drops of *BLEND* in your bath. Soak and relax.

## LIFE STYLE

Make a plan to spend your next 'period week' in a very relaxed fashion.

For instance – get a really interesting book from the library and plan some peaceful evenings curled up on a comfortable sofa with your book and some relaxing music.

Or dig out your favourite video and buy in your favourite menu and plan an evening of relaxed viewing.

Whatever you choose the whole idea is to spoil yourself and let the rest of the world take care of itself for a few days.

## DIET

Drink plenty of spring water.

Keep to a light and easily digestible foods during the period days.

Evening Primrose Tablets as per container.

# Periods – pmt

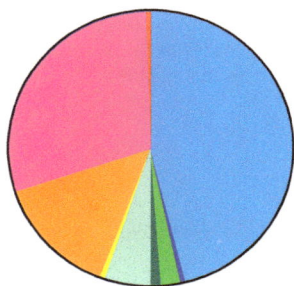

| | | |
|---|---|---|
| 🟦 | esters | 46.0% |
| 🟦 | aliphatic aldehydes | 0.4% |
| 🟦 | ketones | trace |
| 🟩 | sesquiterpenes | 2.4% |
| 🟩 | lactones & coumarins | 1.3% |
| 🟩 | remainder | 5.4% |
| 🟨 | oxides | 0.5% |
| 🟧 | acids | trace |
| 🟫 | aromatic aldehydes | |
| 🟧 | monoterpenes | 14.2% |
| 🟥 | alcohols | 29.4% |
| 🟥 | phenols, phe. ethers | 0.4% |

## CCP of BLEND RECIPE

 🌢🌢 *Clary Sage* (salvia sclarea)

 🌢 *Rose Otto* (rosa damascena)

 🌢 *Bergamot* (citrus bergamia)

*Clary Sage* is calming and a sedative. It helps with panic attacks and depression. It is oestrogen like and should be avoided in cases of hormone related cancers. Recommended for menopausal problems.

*Rose Otto* is balancing, calming and cheering. It increases confidence and is recommended for pmt. It regulates the endocrine system and is hormone like in its action. Believed to release dopamine.

*Bergamot* is antispasmodic and calming. Especially recommended for calming agitation and anxiety. This oil is often the first choice in cases of depression. The aroma is a light, refreshing citrus note. It is used in Earl Grey tea.

*Chemical constituents to be found in the blend may include:*

- 🟦 linalyl acetate, geranyl acetate, neryl acetate, citronellyl acetate
- 🟦 caryophyllenal, citral
- 🟦 thujone, camphor
- 🟩 caryophyllene, germacrene, bourbonene, β-bisabolene
- 🟩 bergaptene
- 🟩 damascenone
- 🟨 1.8-cineole, rose oxide
- 🟧 β-pinene, γ-terpinene, α-terpinene, limonene, stearoptene, camphene
- 🟥 linalool, sclareol, α-terpineol, citronellol, geraniol, farnesol, nerol
- 🟥 methyl hexyl ether, methyl eugenol

## BLEND

| | |
|---|---|
| 20 drops | *Clary Sage* |
| 10 drops | *Rose Otto* |
| <u>10 drops</u> | *Bergamot* |
| <u>40 drops</u> | *BLEND* |

Make up your *BLEND* using the quantities above – store in a small dark glass bottle fitted with a dropper.

## AILMENT

Premenstrual tension – pmt is caused by the change in the balance of female hormones during the menstrual cycle. Troublesome but mainly harmless symptoms become evident in the run up to a period.

Unfortunately this can mean that some women are coping with them for 50% of the month. Problems include fluid retention, swollen joints, food and alcohol cravings, weight gain, skin problems, weakness and headaches. Psychological reactions can manifest themselves in irritability, irrationality, decreased sex drive, insomnia, tearfulness and depression.

The reason for many of the symptoms is the drop in level of progesterone – this in turn causes the sugar and salt levels to rise which will lead to fluid retention. The hormonal balance in the body is a feed back system and it generally restores itself. As fluid retention will affect all the cells in the body including those in the brain this could be the main cause of the problems that arise both physically and mentally. Some women become so disturbed that they literally become another person for a day or two.

## TREATMENT

With a regular cyclic disturbance such as this planning is all important. Try to organise your diary both at work and at home so that during the difficult days you do not attempt unreasonable tasks.

Discuss your problem openly with family and colleagues.

## MASSAGE

Make up a bottle of Periods-pmt Treatment Oil by adding 12 drops of *BLEND* to 30 ml of Almond Oil.

Massage with the Treatment Oil is one of the most effective ways of helping your system balance itself. Massage all around your shoulders where the tension is likely to build up. Also massage your abdomen with circular clockwise strokes and finally massage the small of your back. Do this routine every night starting a fortnight before your period is due.

Book a regular appointment with an aromatherapist who will also be able to personally advise you.

## TISSUES / VAPOURISER

Put drops of *BLEND* on tissues and in your vaporiser as needed.

## BATHS

Put 8 drops of *BLEND* in your baths.

## DIET

Vitamin B6
Evening Primrose Oil

# Post-natal Infections

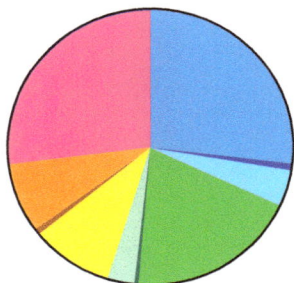

| | | |
|---|---|---|
| ◻ | esters | 27.4% |
| ◼ | aliphatic aldehydes | 0.6% |
| ◻ | ketones | 4.2% |
| ◻ | sesquiterpenes | 19.0% |
| ◼ | lactones & coumarins | 0.2% |
| ◻ | remainder | 3.2% |
| ◻ | oxides | 9.6% |
| ◻ | acids | trace |
| ◻ | aromatic aldehydes | 0.6% |
| ◻ | monoterpenes | 8.2% |
| ◻ | alcohols | 27.0% |
| ◻ | phenols, phe. ethers | trace |

**CCP of BLEND RECIPE**

 *Lavender True* (lavandula angustifolia)

 *Yarrow* (achillea millefolium)

 *Chamomile German* (matricaria recutica)

*Lavender True* is excellent for the regeneration of skin cells. It heals wounds and scars and is on the whole a calming oil. Lower back massage helps dispel afterbirth. It is antiviral, antiseptic and a nervous system regulator.

*Yarrow* acts on the bone marrow and stimulates blood renewal. It is useful for varicose veins, lowers blood pressure and is a good decongestant. The aroma is sweet, spicy and camphorous.

*Chamomile German* is hormone like, temperature reducing and stimulates secretions. It is bactericidal and antiinflammatory – especially helpful for wounds, rashes and skin problems.

*Chemical constituents to be found in the blend may include:*

| | |
|---|---|
| ◻ linalyl acetate, geranyl acetate, lavandulyl acetate, bornyl acetate | ◻ α-bisabolol oxide, 1.8-cineole |
| ◼ citral | ◼ cuminaldehyde, benzaldehyde |
| ◻ isoartemisia, camphor | ◻ α-pinene, β-pinene, sabinene, camphene, ocimene, limonene |
| ◻ chamazulene, caryophyllene, germacrene, dihydroazulene | ◻ terpinen-4-ol, α-terpineol, linalool, borneol, geraniol, lavandulol, α-bisabolol, cadinol |
| ◼ coumarin, umbelliferone, achilline | |
| ◻ en-yn-dicycloether, *cis*-spiro-ether | ◻ eugenol |

## BLEND

| 24 drops | *Lavender True* |
| 8 drops | *Yarrow* |
| 8 drops | *Chamomile German* |
| 40 drops | *BLEND* |

Make up your *BLEND* using the quantities above – store in a small dark glass bottle fitted with a dropper.

## AILMENT

After the birth both mother and baby are adjusting to their new life style. Minor infections are fairly common and nature provides protection to a great extent during the early days. The baby inherits its mother's immunity for a while. In less developed countries mothers use the colostrum that flows from the breasts for 2 to 3 days after birth to heal minor infections. As the colostrum is rich in antibodies just dabbing a little on an infected area can clear infections such as cuts, sores and eye infections.

## BATHS AND BIDETS

After birth the first priority is to keep the genital area scrupulously clean. This will prevent infections from starting up.

If you have a bidet you can use that to fully immerse the genital area.

Otherwise use the bath and just fill to an appropriate level. Add 2 drops of *BLEND* to the bidet and 4 to 8 drops of *BLEND* to the bath depending on the level of water. Also add salt to the water as salt is a natural disinfectant. Use the bidet or bath at least 3 times a day. If you are suffering an infection in the wounds then make sure that you keep the area immersed for at least 5 minutes. This will give the oils time to be absorbed. Don't cheat on this – make the bathroom comfortably warm and rest in the water reading a book.

## TREATMENT

Make up a bottle of Post-natal Treatment Oil by adding 6 drops of *BLEND* to 30 ml of Sweet Almond Oil.

Make up a pot of Post-natal Treatment Lotion by adding 6 drops of *BLEND* to 30 ml of Lotion.

The Treatment Oil and the Treatment Lotion can be used throughout the baby's early months.

If the baby develops any skin rashes or small wounds of any kind just gently apply a little of the oil or lotion. You can also apply the Treatment Oil or Lotion to yourself. If you are experiencing a burning pain on passing urine due to postnatal soreness wash the area and just rub a little Treatment Oil around it. If the pain is really sharp a good trick is to rub a little vaseline on before you urinate. This protects the sore area from the acid in the urine.

Essential oils are excellent for helping skin and wounds to heal.

## DIET

Eat light healthy diet with plenty of fresh vegetables and fruit. Perhaps not too much citrus fruit.

Be careful to keep your calcium level adequate.

# Rheumatoid Arthritis

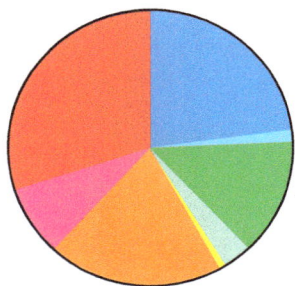

| | | |
|---|---|---|
| ■ | esters | 23.3% |
| ■ | aliphatic aldehydes | trace |
| ■ | ketones | 1.3% |
| ■ | sesquiterpenes | 13.3% |
| ■ | lactones & coumarins | trace |
| ■ | remainder | 2.8% |
| ■ | oxides | 0.8% |
| ■ | acids | trace |
| ■ | aromatic aldehydes | trace |
| ■ | monoterpenes | 20.7% |
| ■ | alcohols | 7.7% |
| ■ | phenols, phe. ethers | 30.1% |

**CCP of BLEND RECIPE**

*Black Pepper* (piper nigrum)

*Clove Bud* (syzygium aromaticum)

*Clary Sage* (salvia sclarea)

*Black Pepper* is analgesic and antispasmodic. It is recommended for aches and pains, rheumatism, rheumatoid arthritis and temporary paralysis. The aroma is sharp and spicy.

*Clove Bud* is analgesic, antispasmodic, an antioxidant and stimulating. It has hormone like properties and balances thyroid problems. The aroma is strong and spicy.

*Clary Sage* is antispasmodic, calming, a sedative and a tonic. It is oestrogen like and should be avoided in cases of hormone related cancers. Do not use if alcohol has been consumed.

---

*Chemical constituents to be found in the blend may include:*

- ■ linalyl acetate, geranyl acetate, neryl acetate
- ■ caryophyllenal
- ■ piperitone, dihydrocarvone, camphor, thujone
- ■ β-caryophyllene, bisabolene, germacrene, bourbonene, humulenes
- ■ 1.8-cineole, caryophyllene oxide
- ■ limonene, α-pinene, β-pinene, sabinene, terpinenes, myrcene, phellandrene, camphene, thujene
- ■ terpinen-4-ol, α-terpineol, linalool, sclareol, α-bisabolol
- ■ myristicin, safrole, aceteugenol, eugenol, methyl hexyl ether

## BLEND

14 drops   *Black Pepper*
14 drops   *Clove Bud*
<u>14 drops</u>   *Clary Sage*
<u>42 drops</u>   *BLEND*

Make up your *BLEND* using the quantities above – store in a small dark glass bottle fitted with a dropper.

## AILMENT

Unlike osteoarthritis which is progressive and irreversible rheumatoid arthritis may come and go spontaneously. There is no sure cure and the underlying causes are not fully understood. Physical and emotional stresses may play some part in triggering an attack. The characteristic feature of an attack is a small knot of inflamed fibrous tissue often just under the skin. Any organ can be affected but the most common are the knuckle joints and the wrist. The inflammation may subside without inflicting much damage but if a chronic attack sets in then the joint may become damaged and eventually deformed. The inflammation causes the muscles around the joint to tighten and the cartilage may become damaged over time.

It is thought that for some reason the immune system sees some normal body cells as 'foreign bodies' and attacks them. Such a disease is classified as an autoimmune disease. Rheumatoid arthritis is more common in women than in men. The pain and inflammation can be helped with the essential oils. Very severe attacks may eventually need surgery to ease the deformities.

As the first attack of the condition often follows a virus infection or an illness it could well be linked to the functioning of the glands and hormones.

## BATHS

Put 2 handfuls of Epsom Salts and 8 drops of *BLEND* in your bath. Bath daily giving yourself time to relax and soak in the comfort of the warm water.

## MASSAGE

Make up a bottle of Rheumatoid Arthritis Treatment Oil by adding 12 drops of *BLEND* to 30 ml of Sweet Almond Oil.

Massage the oil over your shoulders. Get a friend to give you a full body massage or even just a back massage at regular intervals. The oils will be absorbed into your blood stream and will help with the inflammation and pain. Gently apply a little Treatment Oil to affected joints.

## DIET

If you are suffering from severe attacks, it is worth taking some effort to check whether it is a food allergy that is triggering the attacks. If so you may be able to control the condition by following the correct diet.

It is probably best to seek professional help in setting up a closely monitored food plan.

You can try yourself by cutting your diet back to only a few items and then gradually including other items one at a time. You may be able to identify the culprit. Red meat sometimes seems to be the problem.

# Ringworm

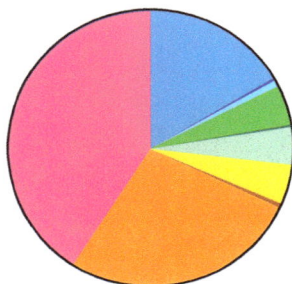

| | | |
|---|---|---|
| | esters | 17.0% |
| | aliphatic aldehydes | 0.2% |
| | ketones | 0.8% |
| | sesquiterpenes | 4.6% |
| | lactones & coumarins | 0.1% |
| | remainder | 3.9% |
| | oxides | 4.6% |
| | acids | trace |
| | aromatic aldehydes | 0.2% |
| | monoterpenes | 27.4% |
| | alcohols | 41.2% |
| | phenols, phe. ethers | trace |

**CCP of BLEND RECIPE**

*Lavender True* (lavandula angustifolia)

*Tea Tree* (melaleuca alternifolia)

*Thyme Common Sweet* (thymus vulgaris linaloliferum)

*Lavender True* is excellent for the regeneration of skin cells. It heals wounds and scars and is on the whole a calming oil. It is recommended for arthritis, burns, radiography burns, eczema, herpes, psoriasis, spots and wounds.

*Tea Tree* is antifungal and strongly antiseptic and is recommended for athlete's foot, bites, boils, burns, radiography burns, cold sores, itching, mouth ulcers, ringworm, spots, sweaty feet, wounds.

*Thyme Common Sweet* is antioxidant, antifungal, antiinflammatory, antiseptic. It is recommended for acne, dry and wet eczema, muscular rheumatism, psoriasis and verrucas.

*Chemical constituents to be found in the blend may include:*

- linalyl acetate, geranyl acetate, lavandulyl acetate
- citral
- octanone, camphor
- aromadendrene, viridiflorene, cadinene, β-caryophyllene
- coumarin, umbelliferone
- 1.8-cineole, linalool oxide
- cuminaldehyde, benzaldehyde
- α-pinene, α-terpinene, γ-terpinene, p-cymene, limonene, terpinolene, myrcene, ocimene, camphene
- terpinen-4-ol, α-terpineol, linalool, borneol, lavandulol, globulol, viridiflorol

## BLEND

| | |
|---|---|
| 8 drops | *Lavender True* |
| 24 drops | *Tea Tree* |
| 8 drops | *Thyme Common Sweet* |
| 40 drops | *BLEND* |

Make up your *BLEND* using the quantities above – store in a small dark glass bottle fitted with a dropper.

## AILMENT

Ringworm is one of the commonest skin diseases. The outer layer of the skin is infected with a microscopic fungus. Athlete's foot is one example of a strain of this fungus. With some types the fungus spreads out as a disc across the skin. The skin in the centre of the disc heals and the fungus moves outwards on the perimeter. This 'ring' appearance gives the condition its name. It can appear on the scalp, in the groin or as mentioned above on the feet. It can also appear elsewhere on the body. If small blisters occur this is an allergic reaction to the fungus. The nails of the fingers and the toes may harbour the fungus which causes them to become slightly deformed. If the fungus is in the scalp small areas of hair loss will be experienced. The fungus can be passed on from people and animals.

## LIFE STYLE

Keep all towels and flannels isolated to prevent the infection spreading. If clothes have been in contact with the fungus add 4 drops of *BLEND* to the rinse water when you wash them. In a washing machine add 4 drops of *BLEND* to the softener that you use for the rinse cycle.

In the case of Athlete's foot avoid changing rooms and swimming pools until the condition has cleared.

## APPLICATION

Apply 1 drop of *BLEND* to the affected area 3 times a day until it is clear. This should take about 10 days. Make up a bottle of Ringworm Treatment Oil by adding 12 drops of *BLEND* to 30 ml of Sweet Almond Oil.

After the fungus has cleared rub the Treatment Oil over the area where the infection was and this will stop it from starting up again. Do this daily for a week.

Watch out for any sign of the fungus returning and repeat the treatment immediately before it has a chance to become established.

# Sex Drive Problems

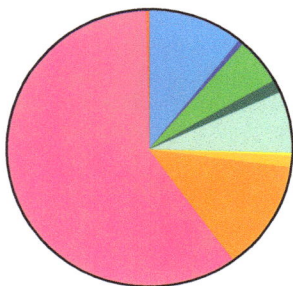

| | | |
|---|---|---|
| | esters | 11.0% |
| | aliphatic aldehydes | 0.4% |
| | ketones | trace |
| | sesquiterpenes | 5.4% |
| | lactones & coumarins | 1.3% |
| | remainder | 7.6% |
| | oxides | 0.1% |
| | acids | 1.3% |
| | aromatic aldehydes | |
| | monoterpenes | 13.2% |
| | alcohols | 59.4% |
| | phenols, phe. ethers | 0.3% |

**CCP of BLEND RECIPE**

*Sandalwood* (santalum album)

*Rose Otto* (rosa damascena)

*Bergamot* (citrus bergamia)

*Sandalwood* is an aphrodisiac, calming and a tonic. It is recommended for impotence. Well known for bringing peaceful feelings – it is used for incenses and meditation.

*Rose Otto* is an aphrodisiac, antispasmodic, balancing and calming. It calms jealous feelings and increases confidence. It is recommended for frigidity and impotence.

*Bergamot* is widely used to calm agitation and panic attacks. It has a gentle action covering a wide range of therapeutic uses. The aroma is light and citrus which balances the rose and sandalwood aromas well.

*Chemical constituents to be found in the blend may include:*

- citronellyl acetate, geranyl acetate, neryl acetate, linalyl acetate
- citral
- santalone
- santalenes, curcumenes, farnesene, caryophyllene, β-bisabolene
- bergaptene
- damascenone
- rose oxide
- nortricycloekasantalic acid
- β-pinene, γ-terpinene, α-terpinene, limonene, stearoptene, camphene
- santalols, tricycloekasantalol, nerol, borneol, citronellol, geraniol, linalool, farnesol
- methyl eugenol

## BLEND

20 drops   *Sandalwood*
10 drops   *Rose Otto*
10 drops   *Bergamot*
40 drops   *BLEND*

Make up your *BLEND* using the quantities above – store in a small dark glass bottle fitted with a dropper.

## AILMENT

Inadequacy, real or imaginary is the commonest reason why people find their sex drive diminished. Frigidity is a lack of sexual desire that is normally applied to women but can equally apply to men. It is important to identify any physical conditions that prevent coitus. A man may be impotent either because he physically cannot achieve an erection due to some physical illness or because of emotional problems.

Sexual activity is usually depressed by general ill health anyway.

Most impotency and frigidity problems are caused by emotional states of mind. Lack of sex drive, rather than being due to any deep seated psychological childhood trauma, is often due simply to a shyness that either sex can suffer from, together with an inferiority complex about their sexual attractiveness. It is seldom that they find their partner sexually unattractive but more likely that they are discontent with their own physical appearance. Unfortunately, their partner can easily misunderstand the problem and feel unnecessarily rejected. In such a case a vicious circle of misunderstanding can set up between the partners.

A woman is seldom roused as quickly as a man and as in nature an initial reluctance is part of the wooing process. Few couple achieve sexual harmony at once, although this is rarely admitted. Patience and understanding are essential ingredients in building a satisfying sexual relationship.

## TREATMENT

Talk through any problem with your partner. Recognise each other's needs and work together to resolve any hang ups. A warm and cosy atmosphere and plenty of time to build up to a climax will provide satisfaction to both partners.

## MASSAGE

Make up a bottle of Sex Drive Problems Treatment Oil by adding 12 drops of *BLEND* to 30 ml of Sweet Almond Oil.

Quite separate from sexual encounters exchange body massages with your partner regularly. Such a massage should not be seeking any sexual response. It is essential that the partner receiving the massage can completely relax rather than be expected to make any response. The aim of the massage is to relax the mind and to create emotional confidence. The essential oils will lower feelings of anxiety and enhance feelings of self esteem.

## VAPOURISER

Put 8 drops of *BLEND* in the vapouriser to create a relaxed environment.

# Sprains

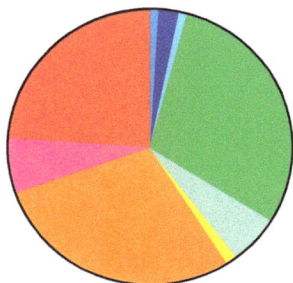

| | | |
|---|---|---|
| ■ | esters | 1.0% |
| ■ | aliphatic aldehydes | 2.5% |
| ■ | ketones | 1.0% |
| ■ | sesquiterpenes | 29.3% |
| ■ | lactones & coumarins | |
| ■ | remainder | 5.6% |
| ■ | oxides | 1.4% |
| ■ | acids | trace |
| ■ | aromatic aldehydes | |
| ■ | monoterpenes | 28.8% |
| ■ | alcohols | 6.4% |
| ■ | phenols, phe. ethers | 24.0% |

**CCP of BLEND RECIPE**

*Ginger* (zingiber officinale)

*Nutmeg* (myristica fragrans)

*Clove Bud* (syzygium aromaticum)

*Ginger* is analgesic and it helps to disperse blood clots. It is a warming oil that stimulates the blood circulation. The aroma is warm, pleasant and spicy. Used in many ancient remedies.

*Nutmeg* is invigorating to heart and circulation. Treat with care the myristicin can cause hallucinations. Avoid in pregnancy.

*Clove Bud* is analgesic, antispasmodic and stimulating. It raises blood pressure. Check for skin irritation. Used in traditional medicine for alleviating toothache. Used in many modern pharmaceuticals. The aroma is strong and spicy.

*Chemical constituents to be found in the blend may include:*

■ geranial, citronellal

■ gingerone

■ β-sesquiphellandrene, zingiberene, *ar*-curcumene, β-caryophyllene, humulenes

■ 1.8-cineole, caryophyllene oxide, humulene oxide

■ α-pinene, β-pinene, α-terpinene, γ-terpinene, sabinene, myrcene, limonene, camphene, *p*-cymene

■ citronellol, linalool, terpinen-4-ol, borneol, gingerol, geraniol

■ eugenol, isoeugenol, aceteugenol, myristicin, elemicin, safrole

## BLEND

| | |
|---|---|
| 20 drops | *Ginger* |
| 10 drops | *Nutmeg* |
| 10 drops | *Clove Bud* |
| 40 drops | *BLEND* |

Make up your *BLEND* using the quantities above – store in a small dark glass bottle fitted with a dropper.

## AILMENT

A sprain occurs when the fibres of the connective tissue are torn and damaged without a bone being broken or dislocated. Sometimes bleeding occurs. The damaged tissue causes swelling and is extremely painful. The body restricts the movement of the area because of the pain and this generally ensures that the movement is reduced such that the healing can take place. This is in contrast to the case of a broken bone which requires setting and plastering. If the pain and swelling from a suspected sprain does not disperse after a day or two there could well be a small fracture in the bone and it is wise to have the injury examined and scanned.

It is possible to sprain or strain any area of the body.

The treatment of a sprain with compresses will speed the recovery in most cases.

Rest the injury as far as possible.

## COMPRESSES

For most sprains the following treatment is recommended. Prepare an ice cold bowl of water and add 5 drops of the BLEND. Make a compress out of clean cotton cloth. Soak the cloth in the prepared water, wring out and place around the injured area. Repeat this several times to start the cooling process and to allow the oils to penetrate the wound. Next use an icebag or even a 'frozen bag of peas' and place it on

the injured area for twenty minutes. Once the swelling subsides and certainly by the next day you can start applying hot and cold compresses alternately. This will encourage the blood to circulate to the injured area and speed up the healing processes.

## APPLICATION

Make up a bottle of Sprain Treatment Oil by adding 12 drops of *BLEND* to 30 ml of Almond Oil.

Just after the injury has occurred gently stroke the Treatment Oil around the area. As the sprain heals you can gradually increase pressure of the strokes. Again you want to encourage blood flow to the injury which together with the oils will speed the healing.

Sprains can take some time to completely heal, a period of 6 to 8 weeks is to be expected.

## BATHS

Put 8 drops of *BLEND*. in your bath. Soak and relax in a warm bath to ease the pain.

# Stretch Marks

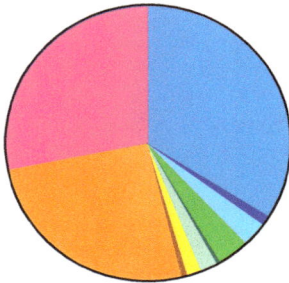

| | | |
|---|---|---|
| | esters | 34.0% |
| | aliphatic aldehydes | 1.0% |
| | ketones | 3.0% |
| | sesquiterpenes | 3.8% |
| | lactones & coumarins | 0.2% |
| | remainder | 2.0% |
| | oxides | 1.5% |
| | acids | |
| | aromatic aldehydes | 0.8% |
| | monoterpenes | 25.5% |
| | alcohols | 28.2% |
| | phenols, phe. ethers | trace |

## CCP of BLEND RECIPE

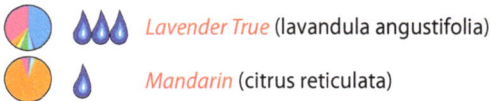

 *Lavender True* (lavandula angustifolia)

 *Mandarin* (citrus reticulata)

*Lavender True* is antifungal, antiinflammatory, antiseptic, a good cell regenerator. It is recommended for all kinds of skin damage such as stretch marks, burns, radiography burns, eczema, herpes, psoriasis, spots, wounds. The aroma is the comfortingly familiar lavender scent with its memories of warm summer days.

*Mandarin* is antiseptic, a cell regenerator and excellent for preventing stretch marks. It acts on the endocrine system and is particularly useful in balancing the metabolic rate. The oil is calming and helps to break down fats, decrease flatulence and improve bile production. This fruit was given to the Mandarins as a mark of respect – hence its name. The aroma is sweet sharp and floral.

---

*Chemical constituents to be found in the blend may include:*

- linalyl acetate, geranyl acetate, lavandulyl acetate, methyl anthranilate
- decanal, sinensal, citral, citronellal
- octanone, camphor
- β-caryophyllene
- coumarin, umbelliferone
- 1.8-cineole, linalool oxide

- cuminaldehyde, benzaldehyde
- γ-terpinene, limonene, pinenes, myrcene, *p*-cymene, ocimene
- linalool, geraniol, terpinen-4-ol, α-terpineol, lavandulol,, citronellol, octanol, borneol
- eugenol, thymol

## BLEND

| | |
|---|---|
| 30 drops | *Lavender True* |
| <u>10 drops</u> | *Mandarin* |
| <u>40 drops</u> | *BLEND* |

Make up your *BLEND* using the quantities above – store in a small dark glass bottle fitted with a dropper.

## AILMENT

If the skin is stretched over long periods it loses some of its elasticity. This results in white silvery stretch marks appearing across the surface of the skin.

In pregnancy the areas at risk of stretch marks are the lower abdomen and the breasts. In adolescence many girls put on extra weight and stretch marks might show up on the thighs and breasts. Obesity of course will also cause this problem to occur. Essential oils cannot cure the damage once it has occurred but they can help the skin's appearance. By far the best approach is to take preventative measures against the forming of stretch marks.

The preventative treatment below will ensure that you do not develop stretch marks during pregnancy.

## MASSAGE

Make up a bottle of Stretch Marks Treatment Oil by adding 12 drops of *BLEND* to 15 ml of Sweet Almond Oil and 15 ml of Calendula Oil.

To keep the skin in excellent condition during pregnancy apply the Treatment Oil to the lower abdomen and around the breasts every evening and morning. Start early in the pregnancy and certainly no later than the fourth month.

## TREATMENT

For skin that is already damaged apply the Treatment Oil every day to improve the condition of the skin. If the stretch marks are due to being overweight do make every effort to tackle the problem. Consider joining a local slimming group such as Weight Watchers. Such a support group can help you with sensible food plans and the help of others who will understand how you are feeling.

## ESSENTIAL OILS

Other essential oils that you can use for stretch marks are:

*Frankincense* (boswellia carteri)
*Myrrh* (commiphora molmol)
*Geranium* (perlargonium graveolens).

# Thrush

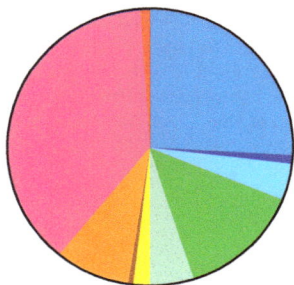

| | | |
|---|---|---|
| ■ | esters | 25.7% |
| ■ | aliphatic aldehydes | 1.1% |
| ■ | ketones | 4.0% |
| ■ | sesquiterpenes | 14.9% |
| ■ | lactones & coumarins | 0.2% |
| ■ | remainder | 4.0% |
| ■ | oxides | 2.1% |
| ■ | acids | trace |
| ■ | aromatic aldehydes | 0.6% |
| ■ | monoterpenes | 8.1% |
| ■ | alcohols | 38.4% |
| ■ | phenols, phe. ethers | 0.9% |

**CCP of BLEND RECIPE**

 *Lavender True* (lavandula angustifolia)

 *Tea Tree* (melaleuca alternifolia)

 *Myrrh* (commiphora myrrha)

*Lavender True* is antifungal, antiinflammatory, antiseptic and an excellent cell regenerator. It is recommended for arthritis, burns, radiography burns, eczema, herpes, psoriasis, spots and wounds. It is generally a calming oil with excellent bactericidal and antiinflammatory properties.

*Tea Tree* is antifungal, antiinflammatory, strongly antiseptic and a parasiticide. It is recommended for athlete's foot, bites, boils, burns, radiography burns, cold sores, itching, mouth ulcers, ringworm, spots, sweaty feet and wounds.

*Myrrh* is bactericidal and antifungal. It has a good drying effect on the skin. It will help the skin heal and also is calming to the nervous system.

*Chemical constituents to be found in the blend may include:*

- ■ linalyl acetate, geranyl acetate, lavandulyl acetate, myrrholic ester
- ■ citral, 2-butanal
- ■ octanone, camphor, curzerenone, methyl isobutyl ketone
- ■ aromadendrene, viridiflorene, cadinene, caryophyllene, elemene, heerabolene, cadinene, copaene
- ■ coumarin, umbelliferone

- ■ 1.8-cineole, linalool oxide
- ■ myrrholic acid
- ■ cinnamaldehyde, cuminaldehyde
- ■ α-pinene, α-terpinene, γ-terpinene, p-cymene, limonene, terpinolene, myrcene, ocimene, camphene
- ■ terpinen-4-ol, α-terpineol, linalool, borneol, myrrh alcohols lavandulol
- ■ eugenol

## BLEND

24 drops   *Lavender True*
 6 drops   *Tea Tree*
12 drops   *Myrrh*
42 drops   *BLEND*

Make up your *BLEND* using the quantities above – store in a small dark glass bottle fitted with a dropper.

## AILMENT

Thrush is an infection that commonly occurs in the mouth, intestines and vagina. It is triggered when the normal level of candida in the body is exceeded. Candida is a fungus related to the yeasts and is a normal part of the body's mucous membranes. If the general bacterial balance of the body is maintained, then the growth of candida is suppressed to the correct level. If the bacterial level is reduced, say by a course of antibiotics, then the level of candida will increase and an attack of thrush may result.

In the mouth thrush can be recognised as white patches. In the vagina it can become quite troublesome and uncomfortable. The area will become itchy and sore and a thick white discharge may set up. The infection can be passed by a sexual partner and once it occurs both partners need to take steps to prevent further outbreaks or it can pass back and forth between them. Overweight people may also be prone to the condition as it settles in warm moist folds of the body. Babies also show the infection in their mouths and in an attack of nappy rash.

## MOUTH WASH

For oral thrush put 1 drop of *BLEND* in a glass of warm boiled water, swish round well. Use as a mouth wash 3 times a day.

## APPLICATION

For vaginal thrush take a tampon and dampen it then place 3 drops of *BLEND* on it and insert in the vagina for 2 hours.

Make up a bottle of Thrush Treatment Oil by adding 12 drops of *BLEND* to 30 ml of Sweet Almond Oil. Apply the Treatment Oil night and morning to the affected area. Wear loose cotton pants and avoid wearing tights until the condition has cleared. Men whose sexual partners suffer from thrush should bathe their penis daily in a bowel of water to which 4 drops of *BLEND* have been added.

## LIFE STYLE

Use sanitary pads not tampons for your periods. Don't take antibiotics unless absolutely necessary. Tell your doctor you are prone to thrush. Don't use strong detergents etc.

## BATHS

Put 8 drops of *BLEND* in your bath. Soak and relax.

## DIET

Cut out sugars and starches.
Eat natural yoghourts.
Take Garlic Tablets and Acidophilus as per container.

# Varicose Veins

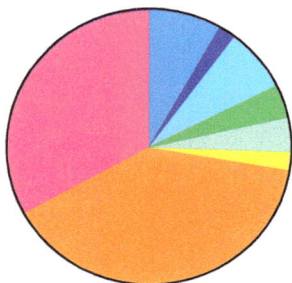

| | | |
|---|---|---|
| ■ | esters | 8.5% |
| ■ | aliphatic aldehydes | 1.7% |
| ■ | ketones | 7.3% |
| ■ | sesquiterpenes | 3.8% |
| ■ | lactones & coumarins | trace |
| ■ | remainder | 4.2% |
| ■ | oxides | 2.3% |
| ■ | acids | trace |
| ■ | aromatic aldehydes | |
| ■ | monoterpenes | 39.2% |
| ■ | alcohols | 33.0% |
| ■ | phenols, phe. ethers | |

**CCP of BLEND RECIPE**

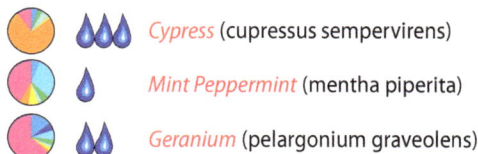

 *Cypress* (cupressus sempervirens)

 *Mint Peppermint* (mentha piperita)

 *Geranium* (pelargonium graveolens)

*Cypress* is astringent, bactericidal and balances the sympathetic nerve system. It constricts blood vessels and is recommended for broken capillaries, cellulite, haemorrhoids, pyorrhoea, rheumatism and sweaty feet.

*Mint Peppermint* antiinflammatory, bactericidal, an analgesic and a tonic to the system. It constricts capillaries and is recommended for asthma, eczema, gnats, herpes, rashes, ringworm and yellow fever.

*Geranium* is anticoagulant, bactericidal and a tonic. It constricts blood vessels, stems bleeding and is recommended for fluid retention and varicose veins. Traditionally a great healing plant often planted around dwellings to ward off evil spirits.

*Chemical constituents to be found in the blend may include:*

■ α-terpinyl acetate, menthyl acetate, citronellyl formate, geranyl formate
■ citral
■ menthone, isomenthone, pulegone
■ guaiazulene, β-caryophyllene, cedrene, cadinene, germacrene
■ aesculetine, menthofuran

■ *cis*-rose oxide, 1.8-cineole
■ α-pinene, β-pinene, Δ3-carene, *p*-cymene, camphene, limonene, phellandrene, menthene
■ cedrol, α-terpineol, borneol, sabinol, manool, menthol, neomenthol, citronellol, geraniol, linalool

## BLEND

| | |
|---|---|
| 21 drops | *Cypress* |
| 7 drops | *Mint Peppermint* |
| <u>14 drops</u> | *Geranium* |
| <u>42 drops</u> | *BLEND* |

Make up your *BLEND* using the quantities above – store in a small dark glass bottle fitted with a dropper.

## AILMENT

This is a painful condition when the veins become distended and knotted. They often show clearly on the surface of the legs and can also form just inside the rectum – see under haemorrhoids.

Obstruction of the blood flow causing pressure on the veins is the cause of the damage. The valves in the veins become damaged and no longer function well. In the legs where the blood is flowing against gravity this results in the veins becoming knotted and distended.

Varicose veins can begin to develop as early as the teenage years. They occur frequently during pregnancy. People whose jobs involve many hours of standing are also at risk of this condition. Obesity also causes strain on the veins.

Phlebitis occurs if veins become inflamed and this sometimes results in a blood clot forming

## TREATMENT

Once the vein is badly damaged it is not possible to repair it. However to help the circulation it is advised to wear support stockings.

Make up a bottle of Varicose Vein Treatment Oil by adding 12 drops of *BLEND* to 30 ml of Sweet Almond Oil.

Apply the Treatment Oil night and morning to the affected area. If working with the leg use strokes from the ankle to the thigh. Always work towards the heart as you are helping the veins send the blood back to the heart. Use the palm of your hand and not your fingers.

## LIFE STYLE

To keep the condition under control avoid standing for long periods. If standing still, to help the blood flow, flex the leg muscles regularly. Take regular exercise. Do not cross your legs when sitting down.

## COMPRESSES

To relieve the aching pain, prepare cold compresses by adding 4 drops of *BLEND* to ice cold water. Use a cotton cloth, soak in the water, wring out and place around the area.

## BATHS

Put 6 drops of *BLEND* in your bath. Soak and relax. Do not have your bath water too hot.

## DIET

If necessary, follow a weight reduction diet.

**Supplements**
Parsley and Garlic
Vitamin C, Vitamin E, Rutin, Lecithin

# Weight Loss

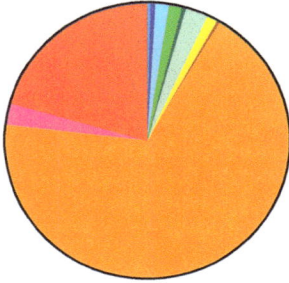

| | | |
|---|---|---|
| ■ | esters | 0.2% |
| ■ | aliphatic aldehydes | 0.6% |
| ■ | ketones | 1.7% |
| ■ | sesquiterpenes | 1.5% |
| ■ | lactones & coumarins | 0.2% |
| ■ | remainder | 3.4% |
| ■ | oxides | 1.0% |
| ■ | acids | trace |
| ■ | aromatic aldehydes | 0.1% |
| ■ | monoterpenes | 68.0% |
| ■ | alcohols | 2.7% |
| ■ | phenols, phe. ethers | 20.6% |

**CCP of BLEND RECIPE**

*Fennel Sweet* (foeniculum vulgare)

*Juniper Berry* (juniperus communis)

*Grapefruit* (citrus paradisi)

*Fennel Sweet* is a decongestant, antiinflammatory and diuretic. It is recommended for cellulite, dissolves boils and treats swellings, fluid retention, oedema and wrinkles. Avoid in cases of pregnancy or epilepsy.

*Juniper Berry* is diuretic and acts as a regulator. It is recommended for cellulite, fluid retention, obesity, oedema, painful joints, psoriasis, stiffness and it eliminates uric acid from the joints.

*Grapefruit* treats congested skin. It is calming and relieves stress headaches. It generally aids digestion. It is a diuretic and has a general cleansing effect on the body.

*Chemical constituents to be found in the blend may include:*

- ■ geranyl acetate
- ■ citronellal, citral, sinensal
- ■ fenchone
- ■ caryophyllene, cadinene, humulenes, germacrene, cadinene
- ■ umbelliferone, auraptene, limettin, bergaptene, umbelliferone
- ■ 1.8-cineole, caryophyllene oxide
- ■ anisic acid
- ■ anisaldehyde
- ■ α-pinene, α-thujene, γ-terpinene, limonene, myrcene, phellandrene, p-cymene, sabinene, camphene
- ■ fenchol, terpinen-4-ol, α-terpineol, paradisiol, geraniol
- ■ trans-anethole, methyl chavicol

## BLEND

| | |
|---|---|
| 16 drops | *Fennel Sweet* |
| 12 drops | *Juniper Berry* |
| <u>20 drops</u> | *Grapefruit* |
| <u>48 drops</u> | *BLEND* |

Make up your *BLEND* using the quantities above – store in a small dark glass bottle fitted with a dropper.

## AILMENT

Obesity is the condition where the body has stored so much extra fat that health is threatened. Overweight can lead to various conditions such as high blood pressure, poor circulation, diabetes, gall bladder problems, gout, heart disorders, heart attacks and shortened life expectancy.

Over weight is caused by overeating in as much that more calories are being taken in than are being burnt up by the body. To adjust the fat level in the body a controlled food plan and life style need to be undertaken. Sometimes young girls are so driven to reduce weight that they cease to eat at all and are unable to reverse the process. This inability to eat diagnosed as anorexia is an extremely dangerous condition and needs expert advice. Help can be obtained from Maisner Centre for Eating Disorders, P.O. Box 464, Hove, East Sussex BN3 2BN.

## TREATMENT

To tackle the problem of obesity, individual treatment plans need to be developed. People have different metabolic rates which is one factor but emotional, psychological and social pressures all play a part. Seek out a friend or a local slimming group such as Weight Watchers to help you develop your own strategy. You will need to adopt a programme that you can establish as a life-long pattern. Do not go for crash dieting – this can do more harm than good in the long term.

Essential oils can most certainly help to reduce fluid retention and also work on your metabolism and hormonal balance.

## MASSAGE

Food is often turned to as a comfort. Replace it with a full body massage by booking regular appointments with an aromatherapist. They will also counsel you on your progress and provide another support in your strategy to establish a new life style. At home make up a bottle of Weight Loss Treatment Oil by adding 12 drops of *BLEND* to 30 ml of Sweet Almond Oil. Use your Treatment Oil, every day, to massage all around your shoulders and lower back. Get a friend to massage your back regularly.

## BATHS

Put 8 drops of *BLEND* in your bath. Soak and relax.

## DIET

Work out your controlled food plan with advice from an expert.

Always include 8 glasses of spring water a day.

# Bibliography

Beckett, S., *Herbs to Soothe Your Nerves*, Thorsons, 1977.

*British Herbal Pharmacopoeia*, British Herbal Medicine Association, 1983.

Culpeper, N., *Culpeper's Complete Herbal*, W. Foulsham and Co. Ltd, 1952.

Davis, P., *Aromatherapy: An A-Z*, C. W. Daniel, 1988.

Duke, J. A., *Handbook of Medicinal Herbs*, CRC Press, Boca Raton, 1985.

Franchomme, P. and Pénoël, D., *L'Aromathérapie Exactement*, Roger Jollois Edit., 1990.

Franchomme, P., *Livre Quatrième, Eléments de Matière Médicale Aromatique Fondamentale*, Roger Jollois Edit., France, 2001.

Franchomme, P., *Phytoguide I*, International Phytomedical Foundation, La Courtête, France, 1985.

Grieve, M., *A Modern Herbal*, Penguin, 1982.

Grosjean, N., *Aromatherapy from Provence*, C. W. Daniel, 1993.

Guenther, E., *The Essential Oils*, Vol. 1-6., Van Nostrand, New York, 1948.

Jackson, J., *Aromatherapy*, Dorling Kindersley, 1987.

Kroch, A. & C. A., *Guide to the Medicinal Plants of the United States*, Quadrangle, The New York Times Book Co., 1973.

Lautie, R. and Passebecq, A., *Aromatherapy: The Use of Plant Essences for Healing*, Thorsons, 1982.

Lawless, J., *Aromatherapy and the Mind*, Thorsons, 1994.

Lawless, J., *The Encyclopaedia of Essential Oils*, Element Books, 1992.

Lawrence, B. M., *Essential Oils*, Allured Publishing Co., Wheaton, USA, 1978.

Le Strange, R., *A History of Herbal Plants*, Angus and Robertson, 1977.

Lis-Balchin, M., *The Chemistry and Bioactivity of Essential Oils*, Amberwood, 1995.

Mabey, R. (Ed.), *The Complete New Herbal*, Elm Tree Books, London, 1988.

Maury, M., *Marguerite Maury's Guide to Aromatherapy*, C. W. Daniel, 1989.

Metcalfe, J., *Herbs and Aromatherapy*, Webb and Bower, 1989.

Mills, S. Y., *The Essential Book of Herbal Medicine*, Penguin Arkana, Harmonsworth, 1994.

Ody, P., *The Herb Society's Complete Medicinal Herbal*, AbeBooks, 1992.

Percival, A., *Aromatherapy – A Nurse's Guide*, Amberwood, 1991.

Phillips, R., *Wild Flowers of Britain*, Pan, 1977.

Price, S. and Price, L., *Aromatherapy for Health Professionals*, Churchill Livingstone, 1995.

Price, S., *Aromatherapy for Common Ailments*, Gaia Books, 1991.

Price, S., *Aromatherapy Workbook*, Thorsons, 1992.

Ranson, F., *British Herbs*, Penguin, 1949.

Rich, P., *Practical Aromatherapy*, Parragon Book Services, 1994.

Ryman, D., *The Aromatherapy Handbook*, Century, 1984.

Secondi, O., *Handbook of Perfumes and Flavors*, Chemical Publishing Co., New York, 1990.

Sellar, W., *The Directory of Essential Oils*, C. W. Daniel, 1992.

Stead, C., *The Power of Holistic Aromatherapy*, Javelin Books, 1986.

Tisserand, M., *Aromatherapy for Women*, Thorsons, 1990.

Tisserand, M., *Stress: The Aromatic Solution*, Hodder and Stoughton, 1996.

Tisserand, R. and Balacs, T., *Essential Oil Safety, A Guide for Health Care Professionals*, Churchill Livingstone, 1995.

Valnet, J., *The Practice of Aromatherapy*, C. W. Daniel (English Version), 1982.

Westwood, C., *Aromatherapy – A Guide for Home Use*, Amberwood, 1991.

Westwood, C., *Aromatherapy – For Stress Management*, Amberwood, 1991.

Wildwood, C., *Aromatherapy*, Element Books, 1991.

Worwood, V. A., *The Fragrant Mind*, Doubleday, 1990.

Worwood, V. A., *The Fragrant Pharmacy*, Macmillan, 1990.

Wren, R. C., *Potter's New Cyclopedia of Botanical Drugs and Preparations*, C. W. Daniel, 1988.

www.ingramcontent.com/pod-product-compliance
Lightning Source LLC
Chambersburg PA
CBHW052029030426
42337CB00027B/4922